LIVE WELL

A Guide To Healthy Living

Larry Allen

KDP AMAZON

Cover design by: Art Painter
Library of Congress Control Number: 2018675309
Printed in the United States of America

To my beloved sons, Tobi and Olayide Allen:

You are the guiding lights of my life and the reason I passionately seek knowledge about wellness and longevity. My deepest hope is to impart this wisdom to you both so you may lead long, healthy, purposeful lives.

As young men entering your prime, treat your body as the precious gift it is. Fill it with nourishing foods to power your dreams. Move it daily in ways that energise your spirit. Allow it rest when worn, and care for it gently through illness. See vitality as your birthright.

To have strength is to use that strength for good, in big ways and small. Lend your strength to causes greater than yourself. Stand up for justice, practice compassion, and walk in others' shoes. Share your gifts wherever you go.

Laugh often, love wholeheartedly, and know your worth. Though storms will come, anchor yourself in faith. Maintain perspective and integrity when faced with life's complexities.

As your father, it brings me boundless joy to watch you grow into the thoughtful, capable individuals you are becoming. I am endlessly proud. May you embrace the wisdom in these pages, and chart a course for health all the days of your lives.

With all my love,
Dad

In addition, I dedicate this book to readers of all ages seeking to improve their wellbeing. May you find these evidence-based insights instructive in your personal health journeys. Whether you are just starting out or have been immersed in wellness for decades, I hope you discover new perspectives within these chapters to challenge assumptions and expand your knowledge.

To those struggling with health issues, my heart is with you. Stay encouraged. Even small steps matter, so begin where you are able. Focus on progress over perfection. And remember - you are so much more than any diagnosis. You are a complex being of infinite worth.

I extend my heartfelt gratitude to each reader of this book. It is a profound honour, and I am deeply humbled to stand beside you in the sacred quest for our well-being. Let us raise a toast to our collective growth in strength and wisdom as we navigate the years ahead!

INTRODUCTION

Live Well: A Guide To Healthy Living

What does it really mean to live well? In today's busy world, it's easy to get caught up in the rush of daily life and lose sight of what's important for our health and happiness. We run from one activity to the next, work long hours, eat on the go, and don't make time for rest, relationships, and renewal. Over time, this takes a toll on our bodies, minds and spirits. We find ourselves stressed, exhausted, unhealthy and disconnected from the things that bring us joy.

The truth is we all deserve to live well - not just exist, but thrive and flourish. Living well means making our health and wellbeing a priority. It requires being intentional about how we nourish our bodies, stimulate our minds, manage our stress, connect with others, and care for our spirits. This book provides a roadmap for just that.

Within these pages, you'll learn simple yet impactful ways to improve your energy, mood, mental sharpness, resilience, relationships, work-life balance, and sense of meaning and purpose. You'll discover the remarkable power of lifestyle choices like exercise, nutrition, sleep, stress management, and social connection for creating a fulfilling, vibrant life. Small, sustainable changes are the focus - not quick fixes or short-term diets and programs.

Use this book as your guide for living with more intention, balance, and joy. With the practical wisdom and science-based advice it offers, you have all the tools needed to feel your best, pursue your passions, and appreciate each day. The time for living well starts now.

TABLE OF CONTENTS

CHAPTER 1: THE FOUNDATION OF HEALTHY LIVING

A healthy lifestyle provides the foundation for overall wellbeing and longevity. While the specifics of a healthy lifestyle can vary between individuals, there are some core pillars that most experts agree upon:

Nutrition

Eating a nutritious, balanced diet is vital for providing the body with essential macro- and micronutrients it needs to function optimally. A healthy diet emphasises whole, minimally processed foods such as fruits, vegetables, whole grains, lean proteins, legumes, nuts/seeds and healthy fats like olive oil and avocados. Limiting added sugars, saturated fats, refined grains and heavily processed foods also contributes to good health. Staying hydrated by drinking plenty of water is additionally important.

Physical Activity

Regular physical activity has extensive benefits for both physical and mental health. Experts recommend at least 150 minutes per week of moderate activity like brisk walking or 75 minutes of vigorous activity like running. Beyond aerobic exercise, strength training and stretching help build strong muscles and bones and improve flexibility. Even small amounts of movement each day, like taking the stairs, can improve health over the long-term.

Stress Management

Chronic stress can negatively impact nearly every body system, from the cardiovascular system to the immune system and brain. Managing stress through techniques like yoga, meditation, deep breathing, and mindfulness, along with getting adequate sleep and making time for hobbies can counter these effects. Identifying stressors and making lifestyle adjustments can also help reduce stress.

Sleep

Quality sleep is essential for energy, mental sharpness, immune function, emotional regulation and overall health. Adults should aim for 7-9 hours per night. Maintaining a consistent sleep routine by going to bed and waking up at the same time, limiting electronics before bed, and creating a restful sleep environment are some key strategies for getting better sleep.

Other Healthy Habits

Additional lifestyle factors that promote wellbeing include not smoking, moderating alcohol intake, engaging in positive social connections, practising self-care, and attending regular medical checkups.

Adopting healthy daily habits and behaviours provides the foundation for optimal wellbeing, quality of life and longevity. The specific components can be adapted to fit each person's unique needs and circumstances. Small, consistent changes to embrace a healthier lifestyle can yield huge payoffs over time.

NUTRITION: NOURISHING THE BODY FOR OPTIMAL HEALTH AND WELL-BEING

Nutrition forms the cornerstone of a healthy and thriving life. It encompasses the process by which the body assimilates and utilises essential substances, known as nutrients, from the foods we consume. These nutrients, comprising both macronutrients and micronutrients, play pivotal roles in sustaining bodily functions, promoting growth, and safeguarding against various diseases. A balanced, nutritious diet lays the foundation for overall well-being and vitality. This essay delves into the critical aspects of nutrition, emphasising the significance of whole, minimally processed foods while cautioning against the harmful effects of certain dietary components.

Macronutrients: Building Blocks of Life

Macronutrients, comprising carbohydrates, proteins, and fats, constitute the primary sources of energy for the body. Carbohydrates, found abundantly in foods like grains, fruits, and vegetables, serve as the body's preferred energy source. They are broken down into glucose, which fuels cellular activities. Proteins, abundant in sources like lean meats, legumes, and dairy, are essential for tissue repair, enzyme synthesis, and immune function. Fats, derived from sources like avocados, nuts, and olive oil, provide a concentrated source of energy, support cell growth, and aid in the absorption of fat-soluble vitamins.

Micronutrients: Tiny Powerhouses of Health

In addition to macronutrients, micronutrients are equally indispensable for maintaining health. These include vitamins and minerals, which are required in smaller quantities but are no less vital. Vitamins, found in a diverse range of foods, serve as co-factors in enzymatic reactions, aiding various metabolic processes. For example, vitamin C boosts immune function and aids in collagen synthesis, while vitamin D supports bone health and calcium absorption. Minerals, such as calcium, iron, and potassium, are crucial for bone strength, oxygen transport, and electrolyte balance, respectively.

The Wholesome Diet: A Symphony of Colors and Textures

A wholesome, balanced diet places emphasis on consuming whole, minimally processed foods. Fruits and vegetables, adorned in an array of vibrant hues, offer a cornucopia of vitamins, minerals, and antioxidants. They provide the body with essential fibre, aiding in digestion and promoting a feeling of fullness. Whole grains like brown rice, quinoa, and whole wheat bread, rich in complex carbohydrates, release energy gradually, stabilising blood sugar levels and sustaining energy levels. Lean proteins from sources like poultry, fish, and legumes offer a complete spectrum of essential amino acids necessary for growth and repair.

Healthy Fats: Nurturing the Body and Mind

Incorporating healthy fats into the diet is paramount for overall well-being. Olive oil, a cornerstone of the Mediterranean diet, is replete with monounsaturated fats, which support heart health by reducing LDL cholesterol levels. Avocados, a creamy and versatile fruit, boast an abundance of omega-3 fatty acids, promoting brain function and reducing inflammation. Nuts and seeds, packed with essential nutrients and fibre, are wholesome snacks that contribute to satiety and provide a myriad of health benefits.

Steering Clear: The Detrimental Culprits

Conversely, certain dietary components have been linked to adverse health effects. Added sugars, prevalent in sugary beverages, candies, and processed foods, contribute to obesity, insulin resistance, and dental issues. Saturated fats, predominantly found in red meat and high-fat dairy products, can elevate LDL cholesterol levels, increasing the risk of heart disease. Refined grains, stripped of their bran and germ layers, lack essential nutrients and fibre, leading to rapid spikes in blood sugar.

Hydration: The Elixir of Life

While focusing on solid foods is paramount, hydration should not be overlooked. Water constitutes a significant portion of the human body and is involved in various physiological processes. Adequate hydration supports digestion, regulates body temperature, and facilitates the transport of nutrients and oxygen. It is recommended to consume an ample amount of water throughout the day to ensure optimal bodily function.

Conclusion

In conclusion, nutrition is the cornerstone of a healthy and vibrant life. A balanced, nutritious diet, rich in macronutrients and micronutrients from whole, minimally processed foods, is essential for optimal bodily function. Prioritising fruits, vegetables, whole grains, lean proteins, legumes, nuts/seeds, and healthy fats while limiting added sugars, saturated fats, and refined grains is pivotal for maintaining good health. Additionally, staying well-hydrated ensures that bodily processes function optimally. By making informed dietary choices, individuals can lay the foundation for a long, thriving life filled with vitality and well-being.

PHYSICAL ACTIVITY

Physical activity refers to any bodily movement that results in the expenditure of energy. Being regularly physically active has far-reaching positive effects on both physical and mental health. According to experts and public health authorities, adults should aim for at least 150 minutes per week of moderate-intensity physical activity or 75 minutes per week of vigorous activity. Ideally, exercise should involve a combination of cardiovascular conditioning, strength training, flexibility exercises, and everyday activity. Building physical activity into one's daily lifestyle is essential for supporting optimal health and wellbeing.

Cardiovascular or Aerobic Exercise

Aerobic exercise involves continuous rhythmic movements that increase the heart rate and breathing rate. Going for brisk walks, jogging, cycling, swimming, dancing, and jumping rope are some examples of aerobic exercise. This type of exercise improves cardiovascular endurance by strengthening the heart and lungs. It may also aid in weight management, regulating blood sugar and cholesterol levels, improving circulation and reducing inflammation. Regular aerobic activity is associated with a reduced risk of heart disease, stroke, type 2 diabetes, some cancers, and premature death.

The Centers for Disease Control and Prevention (CDC)

recommends aiming for at least 150 minutes per week of moderate-intensity aerobic activity, such as brisk walking, casual bicycling or social dancing. Alternatively, 75 minutes per week of vigorous activity like running, swimming laps, or jumping rope also meets the guidelines. This activity can be broken up into multiple sessions of at least 10 minutes each for accumulated benefit. Increasing the duration or intensity beyond minimum recommendations results in even greater health benefits. Those with chronic conditions should consult their healthcare provider for appropriate exercise programs tailored to their needs.

Muscle-Strengthening Exercise

Along with aerobic conditioning, muscle-strengthening activities are an essential component of a well-rounded fitness program. Strength training involves using resistance, such as bodyweight, free weights, resistance bands, or machines, to intentionally activate and strengthen the muscles. It helps build lean muscle mass, enhance bone density, support metabolism and movement, and improve stability and balance. Strength training just two to three times per week can provide excellent results. Allowing at least 48 hours of rest between sessions for each muscle group supports adequate recovery.

Many strength training exercises require minimal equipment. Bodyweight exercises like pushups, lunges, and squats leverage one's own weight as resistance. Other options include lifting free weights like dumbbells or performing exercises with resistance bands. For those with access, weight machines provide adjustable, concentrated resistance. When first getting started, working with a certified personal trainer or using caution to learn proper form is important for safety and effectiveness. Allowing time for a warm up, cool down, and doing light stretching after strength training sessions helps prevent injury.

Improving Flexibility

Flexibility refers to the range of motion available at a joint. Maintaining good flexibility supports mobility, prevents injury, and improves functionality for daily activities and sports. A flexibility program focuses on gentle, sustained stretching of the major muscle groups. This helps increase suppleness and blood flow. Types of stretching exercises include static stretches where a position is held for 10-30 seconds, and dynamic stretches that involve fluid, controlled movements through a full range of motion.

Dedicate time for full-body stretching at least two to three times per week after warming up. Focus on major muscle groups like the shoulders, chest, arms, back, hips, legs and core. Be sure not to bounce or force a stretch - it should not be painful. Those with limited mobility may benefit from working with a physical therapist to develop a safe, personalised stretching program. Regular stretching can help people stay active and mobile with age.

Lifestyle Activity

While structured exercise is extremely valuable, movement incorporated throughout the day is also important for health. Lifestyle physical activity includes things like taking the stairs, walking or biking instead of driving, doing yardwork, actively playing with kids, and choosing to stand when possible. Small bouts of activity, even just a few minutes, accumulate health benefits over time.

Wearable devices like fitness trackers can help monitor daily activity and provide motivation to move more. A general goal is taking at least 5,000 steps per day. Additionally, reducing sedentary behaviours like prolonged sitting through frequent breaks is beneficial. At work or home, try standing while on the phone or during commercial breaks and setting reminders to get up and walk around periodically. Overall, look for opportunities to incorporate more movement into your regular routine.

The importance of exercise cannot be overstated when it comes to living a long, healthy and fulfilling life. A combination of aerobic activity, strength training, flexibility exercises and an active lifestyle provides whole-body health benefits. The time investment required is well worth the payoff of improved physical and mental wellbeing. Start where you are, do what you can, and build up your fitness level gradually over time. With consistency, moving your body more will become a natural part of everyday living.

STRESS MANAGEMENT: NURTURING RESILIENCE FOR OPTIMAL WELL-BEING

In the fast-paced rhythm of modern life, stress has become an ever-present companion. While acute stress can serve as a natural response to challenges, chronic stress can exact a heavy toll on the body and mind. It permeates nearly every physiological system, from the cardiovascular and immune systems to cognitive function. However, by adopting effective stress management techniques, individuals can fortify their resilience and mitigate the adverse effects of prolonged stress. This essay explores the multifaceted impacts of chronic stress and presents a comprehensive approach to its management through practices like yoga, meditation, deep breathing, mindfulness, quality sleep, and engaging in fulfilling hobbies. Additionally, it underscores the importance of identifying stressors and implementing lifestyle adjustments to foster a harmonious and balanced life.

The Cascade of Effects: Chronic Stress on Body Systems

Chronic stress, characterised by prolonged activation of the body's stress response, can unleash a cascade of detrimental effects on various physiological systems. The cardiovascular system bears a significant brunt, with elevated levels of stress hormones leading to increased heart rate, blood pressure, and heightened risk of heart disease. The immune system, too, suffers; prolonged stress can weaken immune function, making individuals more susceptible to infections and illnesses. Moreover, chronic stress exerts a profound impact on the brain, impairing cognitive function, contributing to anxiety and depression, and even affecting memory and learning abilities.

Yoga: Fusing Movement and Mindfulness

One of the most effective tools in stress management is the practice of yoga. This ancient discipline combines physical postures, breathing exercises, and meditation to promote physical and mental well-being. Through the gentle flow of movements and deliberate focus on breath, yoga helps alleviate physical tension, calm the nervous system, and cultivate a sense of inner peace. Regular practice can lead to improved flexibility, muscle strength, and enhanced body awareness. Additionally, yoga fosters mindfulness—a state of present-moment awareness—which is instrumental in reducing stress and enhancing overall mental clarity.

Meditation: Cultivating Tranquillity Within

Meditation stands as a cornerstone of stress management, offering a profound means to cultivate inner calm and mental clarity. It involves training the mind to focus on the present moment, often through techniques like mindfulness meditation, loving-kindness meditation, or transcendental meditation. Regular meditation practice has been shown to reduce the production of stress hormones, lower blood pressure, and enhance emotional well-being. By fostering a sense of detachment from external stressors, meditation empowers individuals to navigate challenges with greater equanimity.

Deep Breathing: The Rhythmic Ebb and Flow of Serenity

Deep breathing exercises serve as a readily accessible and potent antidote to stress. By consciously regulating the breath, individuals can activate the body's relaxation response, counteracting the heightened arousal associated with chronic stress. Techniques such as diaphragmatic breathing or box breathing encourage slow, deliberate inhalations and exhalations, effectively calming the nervous system. Deep breathing can be practised anywhere, making it a versatile tool for immediate stress relief in any situation.

Mindfulness: Embracing the Present Moment

Mindfulness, the practice of non-judgmental awareness of the present moment, offers a transformative approach to stress management. It involves tuning into sensations, thoughts, and emotions without attachment or aversion. By cultivating mindfulness, individuals can develop a heightened capacity to respond to stressors with composure and clarity. This practice not only reduces reactivity but also fosters a greater sense of acceptance and self-compassion.

The Crucial Role of Sleep: Rejuvenating the Mind and Body

Quality sleep stands as an indispensable pillar of stress management. Adequate restorative sleep allows the body to repair and regenerate, bolstering resilience in the face of stressors. Establishing a consistent sleep routine, creating a conducive sleep environment, and practising relaxation techniques before bedtime are crucial steps in promoting restful sleep. Prioritising sleep hygiene contributes significantly to overall well-being and fortifies the body's ability to cope with stress.

Hobbies: Nourishing the Soul

Engaging in fulfilling hobbies provides a meaningful counterbalance to the demands of daily life. Hobbies offer an avenue for creative expression, leisure, and a break from routine stressors. Whether it be painting, hiking, playing a musical instrument, or gardening, investing time in activities that bring joy and fulfilment can serve as a powerful buffer against chronic stress.

Conclusion

In conclusion, chronic stress poses a significant threat to overall well-being, impacting various body systems and cognitive function. However, by adopting effective stress management techniques, individuals can cultivate resilience and mitigate these detrimental effects. Practices like yoga, meditation, deep breathing, and mindfulness offer powerful tools for navigating stress. Additionally, prioritising quality sleep and engaging in fulfilling hobbies contribute to a holistic approach to stress management. Identifying stressors and making lifestyle adjustments further empower individuals to lead balanced, harmonious lives. Through these intentional practices, individuals can nurture their physical, mental, and emotional well-being, fostering a foundation for a thriving and resilient life.

SLEEP

Sleep serves vital restorative functions that are essential for physical health, mental sharpness, emotional regulation, and even longevity. Yet many people struggle with disrupted sleep and poor sleep quality due to factors like work demands, stress, health conditions, and modern technology. Taking steps to consistently get sufficient high-quality sleep is foundational to overall health. Along with proper rest, adopting other positive lifestyle habits also promotes wellbeing.

The Importance Of Adequate Sleep

Experts recommend adults aim for 7-9 hours of sleep per night on a regular basis to allow the body to fully restore and reset. Teenagers require even more, around 8-10 hours. Younger children need 9-12 hours. Sleep has a major impact on nearly every body system:

Immune function relies heavily on sleep, hence the link between sleep deficits and increased sickness.

Sleep is crucial for memory, learning and cognitive performance. Insufficient sleep impairs focus, productivity, decision making, and reaction time.

Metabolic processes including appetite regulation and hormone balance depend on regular sleep cycles. Disruption can promote weight gain and diabetes risk.

Insomnia and sleep apnea increase the risk for cardiovascular disease, stroke, and other heart issues.

Sleep allows the body's repair mechanisms to heal cells and prevents the accumulation of damaging free radicals. Ongoing lack of sleep accelerates biological ageing.

Mental health conditions including depression, anxiety, and substance abuse are exacerbated by poor sleep. Healthy sleep helps maintain stable moods.

Tips For Better Sleep

Many simple changes to daily routines and the sleep environment can have profound impacts on improving sleep duration and quality:

Maintain a consistent sleep schedule, even on weekends. KeepingWake-up and bedtimes within 1-2 hours daily stabilises the circadian rhythm for better rest.

Limit exposure to artificial blue light for 1-2 hours before bed from TV, phones, tablets, and computers. Blue light suppresses melatonin secretion.

Keep the bedroom completely dark, cool, and free of disruptive lights or noises to establish an optimal sleep environment. Consider using an eye mask and earplugs.

Avoid consuming caffeinated drinks after 2pm or heavily drinking alcohol before bedtime. Both interfere with the sleep cycle.

Establish a relaxing pre-bed routine, like reading, gentle yoga, or taking a bath, to transition into sleep. Practising mindfulness or light meditation can also help quiet the mind.

Go to bed when sleepy to avoid tossing and turning. If unable to fall asleep after 20 minutes or you wake up in the night, get up and try a restful activity until drowsy again.

Consider cognitive-behavioural therapy techniques to address habitual insomnia related to thoughts, feelings, behaviours that disrupt sleep.

Beyond proper rest, other healthy lifestyle habits also contribute greatly to wellbeing.

Nutrition Recommendations

Following basic yet essential dietary guidelines lays the foundation for good health:

- Eat a balanced diet rich in whole, minimally processed foods like fruits, veggies, whole grains, lean proteins, healthy fats and legumes. Limit sweets, salty snacks, refined carbs, and saturated/trans fats.

- Stay well hydrated by drinking water and unsweetened fluids regularly throughout the day. Avoid excess sugary or alcoholic beverages.

- Consume a moderate, nutritious breakfast everyday to avoid energy crashes later. Eggs, whole grain toast, fruit, yogurt and nut butter supply sustained energy.

- Fill half your plate with fruits/vegetables to increase fibre, vitamin, mineral and antioxidant intake.

- Choose healthy fats like olive oil and nuts instead of butter, crisco or bottled dressings high in trans fats.

- Read nutrition labels to be aware of portion sizes, added

sugars/sodium, and ingredients in packaged foods. Focus on whole food options when possible.

- Cook at home as often as possible to control ingredients. Meal prep is helpful for making healthy choices despite a busy schedule.

- Allow occasional indulgences in moderation by applying the 80/20 rule - eating nutritious 80% of the time and less healthy 20% of the time.

- Developing Healthy Habits

- In addition to proper nutrition and sleep, adopting other positive lifestyle habits promotes wellbeing:

- Stay mentally sharp by continually learning, reading, playing intellectually engaging games, and trying mentally challenging hobbies.

- Foster personal relationships by connecting regularly with close family and friends. Join groups related to hobbies or volunteer work to expand your social circle.

- Find an exercise regimen you enjoy and stick with it consistently, even starting with just 30 minutes 2-3 times a week. Walking is one of the simplest yet effective forms of exercise.

- Avoid smoking products and excessive alcohol intake, which can jeopardise health in many ways. Seek support in quitting unhealthy addictions.

- Manage stress through healthy outlets like breathing exercises, meditation, yoga, massage, counselling, spending time in nature and participating in recreational activities.

- Develop a sense of purpose and contribute to causes greater than yourself through civic participation, charity work or mentoring others. Altruism is linked to better mental and physical health.

- Make time for fun hobbies that bring you joy, whether gardening, dancing, birdwatching, bowling, or any activity you find fulfilling.

Adopting a lifestyle that includes proper rest, nutrition, exercise, stress management, positive relationships, learning, and purposeful hobbies provides the foundation for optimal wellbeing. When basic healthy habits become ingrained, achieving long-lasting health and life satisfaction becomes second nature.

CHAPTER 2: EATING FOR WELLNESS

Eating a nutritious, well-balanced diet is essential for providing the body with the full range of macro- and micronutrients it needs to function optimally. A healthy diet emphasises whole, unprocessed foods such as fruits, vegetables, whole grains, lean proteins, legumes, nuts/seeds and healthy fats. Limiting added sugars, saturated fats, refined grains and heavily processed foods also contributes to overall wellness.

Macronutrients - Carbohydrates, Protein and Fats

The three major macronutrients that provide energy and calories in food are carbohydrates, protein and fats. Carbohydrates should make up 45-65% of total calories. Focus on whole food sources like fruits, vegetables, whole grains and legumes. Limit added sugars. Protein should be 10-35% of calories, with emphasis on lean animal proteins like poultry, fish, eggs and low-fat dairy as well as plant-based proteins like beans, lentils, nuts and seeds. Dietary fats should make up 20-35% of total calories, with an emphasis on heart-healthy unsaturated fats like olive oil, nuts and avocados rather than saturated animal fats or trans fats.

Incorporate Nutrient-Dense Whole Foods

- Fruits and vegetables provide essential vitamins, minerals, fibre, antioxidants and phytonutrients. Aim for 4-5 servings of veggies and 3-4 servings of fruit daily. Go for a colourful variety.

- Whole grains like oats, brown rice, whole wheat pasta and ancient grains offer important fibre, B vitamins, iron and magnesium with less processing than refined grains.

- Beans and legumes are excellent plant-based protein sources, provide fibre and contain beneficial phytochemicals. Lentils, chickpeas and all varieties of beans are good choices.

- Nuts and seeds offer healthy unsaturated fats along with protein, fibre and micronutrients. They make a satisfying snack in moderation.

Adequate Hydration

Drinking enough water and limiting sugary beverages is vital for health. Aim for 64 ounces (8 cups) of total fluids daily as a general guideline. Thirst is also an indicator of hydration needs. Water helps transport nutrients, removes wastes and protects tissues and organs.

Developing Healthy Eating Patterns

Creating balanced, enjoyable eating patterns is key for a healthy diet, rather than restrictive rules or regimes. Fill half your plate with fruits/vegetables, a quarter with lean protein and a quarter with whole grains at meals. Read nutrition labels and know how to identify healthy choices within each food group. Allow room for occasional treats in moderation without guilt. Making gradual changes and developing sustainable habits leads to lasting improvement.

Overall, emphasising whole, minimally processed foods within a balanced diet contributes to optimal nutritional wellbeing and forms the foundation for good health.

MACRONUTRIENTS: THE CORNERSTONES OF A BALANCED DIET

Macronutrients form the fundamental building blocks of our diet, providing the energy and essential components necessary for bodily functions. Carbohydrates, proteins, and fats constitute the trio of macronutrients, each playing a distinct role in sustaining life and supporting optimal health. This essay explores the significance of these macronutrients, delving into their recommended proportions in a balanced diet and highlighting the importance of choosing wholesome sources for each.

Carbohydrates: Fueling the Body's Engine

Carbohydrates, often referred to as the body's primary source of energy, are composed of sugars, starches, and fibre. They are vital for providing quick, accessible energy that fuels the brain, muscles, and other bodily functions. A balanced diet typically recommends that carbohydrates should constitute between 45-65% of total caloric intake. However, the quality of carbohydrates matters significantly. Whole, minimally processed sources like fruits, vegetables, whole grains, and legumes offer a rich array of vitamins, minerals, and fibre, which are essential for maintaining proper digestion, stabilising blood sugar levels, and promoting overall health. In contrast, added sugars found in sugary snacks and beverages should be limited, as excessive consumption can lead to metabolic imbalances and other health issues.

Protein: The Body's Structural Backbone

Proteins are indispensable for the body's growth, repair, and maintenance. They are composed of amino acids, which serve as the building blocks for various tissues, enzymes, hormones, and immune components. A balanced diet recommends that protein should constitute between 10-35% of total caloric intake. Lean animal proteins, such as poultry, fish, eggs, and low-fat dairy, are excellent sources of high-quality protein. They offer a complete spectrum of essential amino acids necessary for optimal bodily function. Plant-based proteins, including beans, lentils, nuts, and seeds, are also rich sources of protein and provide an array of other essential nutrients. Balancing protein intake from both animal and plant sources can contribute to overall health and well-being.

Fats: Essential for Vital Functions

Dietary fats are essential for various bodily functions, including the absorption of fat-soluble vitamins (A, D, E, and K), the formation of cell membranes, and the production of hormones. They also serve as an energy reserve. A balanced diet typically recommends that fats should constitute between 20-35% of total caloric intake. However, the type of fats consumed is crucial. Emphasis should be placed on heart-healthy unsaturated fats, such as those found in olive oil, nuts, and avocados. These fats can help improve cholesterol levels, support cardiovascular health, and reduce inflammation. In contrast, saturated fats, primarily found in animal products, and trans fats, commonly found in processed and fried foods, should be limited due to their association with various health risks.

Choosing Wisely: A Balanced Approach

Achieving a balanced macronutrient intake involves making mindful and informed dietary choices. It is not only about meeting specific percentage recommendations but also about the quality and diversity of the sources. Incorporating a variety of whole, minimally processed foods ensures a broad spectrum of nutrients necessary for optimal health. This includes an array of colourful fruits and vegetables, whole grains like brown rice and quinoa, lean proteins from both animal and plant sources, and healthy fats like olive oil, nuts, and avocados.

The Role of Individual Variation

It's important to acknowledge that individual dietary needs may vary based on factors such as age, activity level, and specific health conditions. Athletes, for instance, may require higher protein intake to support muscle repair and growth. Individuals with certain medical conditions may need to monitor their carbohydrate intake more closely. Consulting with a healthcare provider or registered dietitian can help tailor macronutrient intake to individual needs and goals.

Conclusion: Nourishing the Body, Mind, and Spirit

In conclusion, macronutrients—carbohydrates, proteins, and fats—constitute the backbone of a balanced diet, providing the energy and essential components necessary for bodily functions. Striking the right balance and choosing nutrient-dense sources are paramount for maintaining optimal health and well-being. By emphasising whole, minimally processed foods and being mindful of the quality of fats, individuals can nurture their bodies, supporting not only physical vitality but also mental and emotional well-being. Tailoring macronutrient intake to individual needs ensures a holistic approach to nourishment, laying the foundation for a vibrant and thriving life.

Incorporate Nutrient-Dense Whole Foods For Optimal Health

The foundation of a healthy, balanced diet lies in the incorporation of nutrient-dense whole foods. These natural, minimally processed options are rich in essential vitamins, minerals, fibre, antioxidants, and phytonutrients that are vital for the body's optimal functioning. This essay delves into the key categories of nutrient-dense whole foods, providing recommendations for their daily intake and highlighting their unique benefits.

Fruits and Vegetables: Nature's Nutrient Powerhouses

Fruits and vegetables stand as the cornerstone of a nutritious diet, offering a treasure trove of essential nutrients. They are abundant sources of vitamins, including vitamin C, vitamin A, and various B vitamins, each playing pivotal roles in metabolism, immune function, and overall health. Minerals like potassium, magnesium, and folate are also prevalent, contributing to proper heart function, bone health, and cell division. Moreover, the high fibre content in fruits and vegetables aids in digestion, regulates blood sugar levels, and promotes a feeling of satiety.

To reap the full spectrum of benefits, individuals should aim for a daily intake of 4-5 servings of vegetables and 3-4 servings of fruit. It is advised to embrace a vibrant variety of colours, as different hues signify distinct phytonutrient profiles. For instance, deep greens like spinach and kale are rich in chlorophyll and folate, while red and orange produce like tomatoes and carrots are packed with antioxidants like lycopene and beta-carotene. By incorporating an array of fruits and vegetables into daily meals, individuals can harness the full potential of these nutrient-dense powerhouses.

Whole Grains: The Wholesome Heart of the Plate

Whole grains, in contrast to their refined counterparts, retain their nutrient-rich bran and germ layers. This means they are rich in fibre, B vitamins, iron, and magnesium, offering sustained energy and a wealth of health benefits. Staples like oats, brown rice, whole wheat pasta, and ancient grains like quinoa and farro are excellent choices. The fibre content in whole grains supports healthy digestion, stabilises blood sugar levels, and helps maintain a healthy weight.

Furthermore, B vitamins are crucial for energy metabolism, cognitive function, and the formation of red blood cells. Iron aids in oxygen transport, while magnesium supports muscle function and bone health. By choosing whole grains over refined options, individuals can make a significant contribution to their overall well-being.

Beans and Legumes: Plant-Based Protein Powerhouses

Beans and legumes are stellar additions to a nutrient-dense diet, particularly for individuals seeking plant-based protein sources. They are not only rich in protein but also provide ample fibre, making them an excellent choice for maintaining satiety and supporting digestive health. Additionally, these humble legumes contain beneficial phytochemicals, such as flavonoids and lignans, which contribute to their antioxidant properties.

Lentils, chickpeas, black beans, and a variety of other legumes are versatile options that can be incorporated into a wide range of dishes. They lend themselves well to soups, salads, stews, and even veggie burgers. Regular consumption of beans and legumes can contribute to overall protein intake, making them an essential component of a balanced diet, especially for those following a vegetarian or vegan lifestyle.

Nuts and Seeds: Nature's Nutrient-Dense Snacks

Nuts and seeds are nutritional powerhouses that offer a plethora of health benefits. They are dense in healthy unsaturated fats, which play a crucial role in supporting heart health and reducing inflammation. Additionally, nuts and seeds are excellent sources of protein, making them a satisfying snack option that can help maintain energy levels throughout the day. The presence of fibre, vitamins, and minerals further enhances their nutritional profile.

Options like almonds, walnuts, chia seeds, flaxseeds, and pumpkin seeds provide a diverse array of nutrients. From omega-3 fatty acids for brain health to magnesium for muscle function, these tiny packages offer a concentrated dose of goodness. However, it's important to consume them in moderation, as they are calorie-dense. Incorporating a small handful of nuts or a sprinkle of seeds into meals or snacks can be a simple yet impactful way to boost nutrient intake.

Conclusion: Nourishing the Body with Nature's Bounty

Incorporating nutrient-dense whole foods into one's diet is a cornerstone of optimal health and well-being. Fruits and vegetables, whole grains, beans and legumes, as well as nuts and seeds, offer a wealth of essential nutrients that support bodily functions and promote vitality. By embracing a colourful array of plant-based foods and choosing whole grains over refined options, individuals can harness the full potential of these natural powerhouses. Whether through hearty salads, nourishing grain bowls, or wholesome snacks, integrating these nutrient-dense options into daily meals lays the foundation for a vibrant, thriving life. By prioritising whole, minimally processed foods, individuals empower themselves to take charge of their health and cultivate a foundation for long-term well-being.

Adequate Hydration: Nourishing The Body With Vital Fluids

Water, the elixir of life, forms the bedrock of human health and well-being. Adequate hydration is paramount for the body's optimal functioning, influencing everything from cognitive performance to physical endurance. This essay unravels the crucial importance of maintaining proper hydration levels, offering guidelines for daily fluid intake, and shedding light on the multifaceted roles of water in the body's intricate systems.

The Essence of Hydration

Water, often referred to as the essence of life, is a fundamental component of human physiology. It comprises a significant portion of the human body, contributing to various critical functions. Beyond quenching thirst, water plays a pivotal role in transporting essential nutrients to cells, removing metabolic waste products, and safeguarding delicate tissues and organs from damage. This underscores the irreplaceable significance of maintaining proper hydration levels for overall health and vitality.

Guidelines for Daily Fluid Intake

Establishing a baseline for daily fluid intake is essential for ensuring optimal hydration. A commonly cited guideline recommends consuming 64 ounces, or roughly 8 cups, of total fluids per day. However, it's crucial to recognize that individual hydration needs may vary based on factors such as age, activity level, climate, and overall health. Athletes and individuals engaged in strenuous physical activity may require additional fluids to compensate for increased sweat loss. Likewise, individuals living in hot, arid climates may need to augment their fluid intake to offset higher rates of water evaporation through perspiration.

Listening to Thirst: A Natural Indicator

Thirst stands as the body's innate signal for the need for hydration. It serves as a reliable indicator that prompts individuals to replenish lost fluids. Ignoring thirst cues can lead to mild dehydration, which can manifest as symptoms like dry mouth, dark urine, and fatigue. Chronic dehydration, if left unaddressed, can lead to more severe health issues, including impaired cognitive function, kidney dysfunction, and increased risk of urinary tract infections.

Limiting Sugary Beverages: A Prudent Choice

While fluids are vital for hydration, not all beverages are created equal. Sugary drinks like sodas, fruit juices, and energy drinks can contribute excessive amounts of added sugars to the diet. Excessive sugar consumption is associated with a myriad of health issues, including obesity, type 2 diabetes, and dental problems. Therefore, it's prudent to limit the intake of sugary beverages and opt for healthier alternatives like water, herbal teas, or naturally flavoured infused water.

Water: A Multipurpose Elixir

Beyond its fundamental role in hydration, water exerts a far-reaching influence on various bodily functions. It serves as a solvent, facilitating chemical reactions necessary for metabolism. Water aids in temperature regulation, acting as a coolant through perspiration and evaporative cooling. Furthermore, it acts as a lubricant for joints, protecting against friction and supporting smooth movement. Additionally, water is crucial for the proper functioning of the digestive system, aiding in the breakdown and absorption of nutrients.

Hydration and Cognitive Function

Proper hydration is closely linked to cognitive function. Research has shown that even mild dehydration can impair cognitive performance, affecting aspects of attention, memory, and mood. Studies suggest that maintaining adequate hydration levels can enhance cognitive function, supporting optimal mental acuity and alertness. This underscores the importance of staying well-hydrated, particularly in situations that demand cognitive focus and concentration.

Conclusion: Nurturing Health through Adequate Hydration

In conclusion, adequate hydration is a cornerstone of overall health and well-being. Water plays a multifaceted role in the body, from transporting essential nutrients to protecting vital organs and tissues. Establishing a baseline for daily fluid intake, listening to thirst cues, and choosing hydrating options wisely are crucial steps in maintaining proper hydration levels. By prioritising water and minimising the consumption of sugary beverages, individuals empower themselves to nurture their health and vitality. Recognizing the intricate interplay between hydration and cognitive function further underscores the profound impact of proper fluid intake on overall well-being. Through these intentional practices, individuals pave the way for a life filled with vibrancy, energy, and sustained well-being.

Developing Healthy Eating Patterns: A Sustainable Approach To Nutritional Well-Being

The quest for a healthy diet often leads individuals down various paths, from fad diets to rigid rules and restrictive eating patterns. However, the key to true nutritional well-being lies in the cultivation of balanced, enjoyable eating patterns rather than adhering to stringent regimens. We explore the principles of developing healthy eating habits, emphasising the importance of balance, mindful choices, and sustainable practices. By focusing on whole, minimally processed foods and adopting gradual changes, individuals can establish a foundation for lasting improvement in their overall health and well-being.

Balanced Plates: The Foundation of Nutritional Health

A crucial step in developing healthy eating patterns is to establish balanced meals that provide a diverse array of essential nutrients. The "plate method" serves as a practical guide, encouraging individuals to allocate their meal components effectively. Ideally, half of the plate should be filled with fruits and vegetables, a quarter with lean protein, and the remaining quarter with whole grains.

Fruits and Vegetables: Nature's Nutrient Powerhouses

Fruits and vegetables are veritable treasure troves of essential vitamins, minerals, antioxidants, and fibre. They offer a diverse array of nutrients that support a wide range of bodily functions. Incorporating a colourful variety ensures a broad spectrum of health benefits. Deep greens provide folate and chlorophyll, reds and oranges offer beta-carotene and lycopene, and blues and purples deliver anthocyanins and flavonoids. These natural compounds confer antioxidant properties, aiding in the protection of cells from damage caused by free radicals.

Lean Proteins: Building Blocks for Growth and Repair

Proteins are integral to the body's growth, repair, and maintenance. They are composed of amino acids, which serve as the building blocks for various tissues, enzymes, hormones, and immune components. Incorporating lean protein sources like poultry, fish, lean meats, eggs, and plant-based options like legumes, tofu, and tempeh, ensures a balanced intake of essential amino acids. These nutrients are crucial for muscle development, enzyme synthesis, immune function, and more.

Whole Grains: Nutrient-Dense Energy Sources

Whole grains form an integral part of a balanced diet, providing vital nutrients like fibre, B vitamins, iron, and magnesium. Unlike their refined counterparts, whole grains retain their bran and germ layers, offering sustained energy and a wealth of health benefits. Staples like oats, brown rice, whole wheat pasta, quinoa, and farro are excellent choices. The fibre content in whole grains supports healthy digestion, regulates blood sugar levels, and helps maintain a healthy weight. B vitamins are crucial for energy metabolism, cognitive function, and the formation of red blood cells. Iron aids in oxygen transport, while magnesium supports muscle function and bone health.

Reading Nutrition Labels: Making Informed Choices

Understanding how to read nutrition labels is a powerful tool for making informed choices within each food group. Labels provide essential information about serving sizes, nutrient content, and the presence of additives or allergens. Paying attention to key elements such as calories, macronutrient content (including fats, proteins, and carbohydrates), fibre, and added sugars can help individuals select foods that align with their nutritional goals. Additionally, being aware of ingredient lists can help identify and avoid heavily processed or overly refined products.

Moderation, Not Deprivation: Room for Treats

In the pursuit of healthy eating patterns, it's important to recognize that occasional treats can have a place in a balanced diet. The key lies in moderation and mindful consumption. Enjoying a piece of dark chocolate, a small serving of dessert, or a favourite indulgence on occasion can be a source of pleasure and satisfaction without undermining overall health goals. It's essential to approach treats with a sense of enjoyment and without guilt, understanding that they are part of a holistic approach to nourishment.

Gradual Changes for Lasting Improvement

Embarking on a journey towards healthier eating patterns is most effective when approached with gradual, sustainable changes. Abrupt and drastic shifts in dietary habits can be difficult to maintain over the long term. Instead, focusing on small, manageable adjustments allows individuals to adapt to new eating patterns at a comfortable pace. This could include incorporating an extra serving of vegetables each day, swapping refined grains for whole grains, or trying a new type of lean protein. Over time, these small changes accumulate, leading to significant and lasting improvements in overall health and well-being.

Emphasising Whole, Minimally Processed Foods

At the heart of developing healthy eating patterns lies an emphasis on whole, minimally processed foods. These natural, nutrient-dense options provide a wealth of essential vitamins, minerals, fibre, and antioxidants. They support optimal bodily function, promote sustained energy levels, and contribute to overall well-being. By prioritising whole foods, individuals ensure that their bodies receive the full spectrum of nutrients necessary for optimal health.

Conclusion: Nurturing Well-being through Mindful Nutrition

In conclusion, developing healthy eating patterns is a journey marked by balance, informed choices, and sustainable practices. By adopting a plate method that prioritises fruits, vegetables, lean proteins, and whole grains, individuals lay the foundation for optimal nutritional well-being. Understanding how to read nutrition labels empowers individuals to make informed choices within each food group. Embracing occasional treats in moderation allows for a balanced and enjoyable approach to nourishment. Gradual, sustainable changes lead to lasting improvement, fostering a sense of well-being that transcends the dinner plate.

Ultimately, the emphasis on whole, minimally processed foods forms the bedrock of healthy eating patterns. These nutrient-dense options provide the body with the essential components it needs to function optimally. By making mindful, intentional choices, individuals can nurture their well-being and set the stage for a life filled with vitality and sustained health. Through these practices, individuals embark on a journey towards a nourished, balanced, and thriving existence.

CHAPTER 3: POWERING YOUR BODY THROUGH EXERCISE

Exercise is not merely a physical activity; it's a powerful tool that can transform your body and mind. Regular physical activity comes with a host of benefits that span from enhancing physical health to boosting mental well-being. This comprehensive guide will delve into the numerous advantages of exercise, along with specific recommendations for different types of workouts, including aerobic exercises, strength training, and flexibility routines. Additionally, we'll explore how to initiate and maintain an exercise routine, the importance of setting goals and tracking progress, and strategies for staying motivated throughout your fitness journey.

Benefits of Exercise

Physical Health

1. Improved Cardiovascular Health: Regular exercise strengthens the heart, reducing the risk of heart disease and high blood pressure.

2. Weight Management: Combining exercise with a balanced diet helps in maintaining a healthy weight or losing excess body fat.

3. Enhanced Immune Function: Regular physical activity boosts the immune system, making you more resistant to illnesses and infections.

4. Improved Bone Health: Weight-bearing exercises like walking and strength training help maintain bone density, reducing the risk of osteoporosis.

5. Better Metabolic Health: Exercise improves insulin sensitivity and metabolic rate, reducing the risk of metabolic disorders like type 2 diabetes.

6. Increased Energy Levels: Regular exercise enhances the body's ability to deliver oxygen and nutrients to tissues, increasing overall energy levels.

7. Improved Digestive Health: Physical activity can aid in preventing constipation and promoting regular bowel movements.

8. Better Sleep Quality: Regular exercise helps regulate sleep patterns and promotes deeper, more restful sleep.

Mental and Emotional Well-being

1. Reduced Stress Levels: Exercise triggers the release of endorphins, chemicals in the brain that act as natural painkillers and mood elevators.

2. Improved Mood and Mental Health: Regular exercise is associated with reduced symptoms of depression, anxiety, and stress.

3. Enhanced Cognitive Function: Physical activity improves memory, attention, and overall cognitive function.

4. Increased Confidence and Self-Esteem: Achieving fitness goals can boost self-confidence and improve body image.

5. Better Coping Mechanisms: Regular exercise can provide healthy outlets for managing emotions and stress.

6. Social Interaction: Group activities or team sports offer opportunities for socialisation and building connections.

Aerobic Exercise Recommendations

Aerobic exercises focus on improving cardiovascular health, respiratory function, and endurance. They involve continuous, rhythmic movements that increase heart rate and breathing. Here are some recommendations for effective aerobic exercise:

1. Types of Aerobic Exercise:

- Brisk Walking: A low-impact activity suitable for all fitness levels.

- Running/Jogging: Increases cardiovascular fitness and burns calories efficiently.

- Cycling: Provides a low-impact option that strengthens leg muscles and improves endurance.

- Swimming: Works multiple muscle groups and is gentle on the joints.

- Dancing: Combines fun and fitness, improving coordination and cardiovascular health.

2. Frequency: Aim for at least 150 minutes of moderate-intensity aerobic activity or 75 minutes of vigorous-intensity activity per week.

3. Intensity:

- Moderate Intensity**: You should be able to talk, but not sing, during the activity.

- Vigorous Intensity**: Your heart rate is significantly elevated, and talking is difficult.

4. Warm-up and Cool-down: Always start with a 5-10 minute warm-up and end with a cool-down to gradually transition your body in and out of exercise.

5. Variation: Mix different forms of aerobic exercise to keep your routine interesting and target various muscle groups.

Strength Training Recommendations

Strength training, also known as resistance training, focuses on building muscle strength, tone, and mass. It's crucial for overall physical function and injury prevention. Here are some recommendations for effective strength training:

1. Types of Strength Training:

- Bodyweight Exercises: Push-ups, squats, and planks use your body's own resistance for strength gains.

- Free Weights: Dumbbells, barbells, and kettlebells provide resistance for a wide range of exercises.

- Resistance Bands: Versatile tools that provide resistance during various movements.

- Weight Machines: Target specific muscle groups using guided equipment available in gyms.

2. Frequency: Aim for strength training exercises at least 2-3 times per week, targeting all major muscle groups.

3. Sets and Repetitions:

- For muscle endurance: 2-4 sets of 12-15 repetitions.

- For muscle strength: 3-5 sets of 6-8 repetitions.

4. Progression: Gradually increase the weight or resistance to continually challenge your muscles.

5. Rest Periods: Allow 48 hours of recovery between sessions targeting the same muscle groups.

Stretching and Flexibility Exercises

Flexibility exercises improve the range of motion in your joints and reduce the risk of injury. Incorporate these into your routine:

1. Types of Flexibility Exercises:

- Static Stretching: Hold each stretch for 15-60 seconds, targeting major muscle groups.

- Dynamic Stretching**: Active movements that gently take your joints and muscles through their range of motion.

- Yoga and Pilates: Combines flexibility, strength, and balance exercises.

2. Frequency: Aim to stretch major muscle groups 2-3 times per week, or daily for more advanced practitioners.

3. Warm-up: Perform light aerobic activity before stretching to increase blood flow and warm muscles.

4. Breathing and Relaxation: Focus on deep, rhythmic breathing to enhance the effectiveness of stretching.

5. Avoid Bouncing: Never use bouncing or jerky movements during stretching, as it can lead to muscle strain.

Getting Started with an Exercise Routine

Starting an exercise routine requires careful planning and consideration of your individual needs and preferences. Here are some steps to help you get started:

1. Consult a Healthcare Professional: Especially if you have existing health concerns or medical conditions.

2. Set Realistic Goals: Define specific, achievable objectives that align with your fitness level and lifestyle.

3. Choose Activities You Enjoy: Opt for exercises that you find enjoyable, as this increases the likelihood of long-term adherence.

4. Create a Balanced Routine:

Include a mix of aerobic, strength training, and flexibility exercises for comprehensive fitness.

5. Consider Time and Location: Determine when and where you'll be most likely to engage in physical activity.

6. Start Slow and Gradually Progress: Begin with manageable durations and intensities, then gradually increase.

7. Listen to Your Body: Pay attention to how your body feels during and after exercise. Rest when needed and seek professional advice if you experience discomfort.

Goal Setting and Tracking Progress

Setting clear, measurable goals is instrumental in maintaining motivation and gauging progress. Here's a structured approach to goal setting:

1. Specific Goals: Clearly define what you want to achieve. For example, "I want to run a 5K in under 30 minutes."

2. Measurable Goals: Attach numbers or specific metrics to your goals. This allows for concrete evaluation of progress.

3. Achievable Goals: Ensure that your goals are realistic and attainable within your current circumstances and capabilities.

4. Relevant Goals: Make sure your goals align with your broader

objectives and personal values.

5. Time-Bound Goals: Set a specific timeline for achieving your goals. This creates a sense of urgency and accountability.

6. Track Your Progress: Keep a record of your workouts, noting duration, intensity, and any notable achievements.

7. Adjust and Adapt: Be flexible with your goals and willing to adapt them as needed based on your progress and changing circumstances.

Maintaining Motivation

Sustaining motivation over the long term is essential for a consistent exercise routine. Employ these strategies to stay inspired:

1. Variety: Change your routine regularly to prevent boredom and challenge different muscle groups.

2. Find a Workout Buddy: Exercising with a friend provides accountability and makes workouts more enjoyable.

3. Set New Challenges: Continuously set new goals to keep things fresh and provide a sense of accomplishment.

4. Incorporate Enjoyable Activities: Engage in activities you love, whether it's dancing, hiking, or playing a sport.

5. Reward Yourself: Celebrate your achievements, no matter how small, to reinforce positive behaviour.

6. Visualise Success: Mentally picture yourself achieving your goals to enhance motivation and focus.

7. Seek Professional Guidance**: Consider working with a personal trainer or fitness coach for expert guidance and personalised routines.

Conclusion

Embarking on a journey of physical fitness through exercise is a transformative endeavour. The benefits encompass not only physical health but also mental and emotional well-being. By incorporating a balanced blend of aerobic exercise, strength training, and flexibility routines, individuals can achieve a comprehensive level of fitness. Setting clear goals, tracking progress, and maintaining motivation are essential elements of a successful fitness journey.

Remember, the key to long-term success lies in consistency, enjoyment, and adaptability. Listen to your body, embrace variety, and seek professional guidance when needed. Ultimately, through the power of exercise, you have the opportunity to enhance your quality of life, unlock your potential, and embrace a healthier, more vibrant version of yourself.

CHAPTER 4:
RELIEVING STRESS
FOR BETTER HEALTH

Stress is an inevitable part of life. However, chronic, ongoing stress can negatively impact nearly every system in the body and contribute to numerous health issues. Taking intentional steps to manage stress through lifestyle changes, relaxation practices, and seeking professional help when needed is foundational to overall wellness.

Effects of Chronic Stress on Health

While temporary, acute stress is normal and can even sharpen focus, chronic stress takes a major toll on physical and mental health in several ways:

- Weakens the immune system, increasing susceptibility to colds, flu and infections. Impairs vaccine responses.

- Raises blood pressure, heart rate, and promotes inflammation, exacerbating heart disease, stroke, and hypertension risk.

- Disrupts digestion, which can lead to ulceration, chronic heartburn, diarrhoea or constipation. Impacts appetite.

- Alters brain structure and function. Impairs cognition, memory and mental performance. Linked to dementia risk.

- Triggers depression and anxiety. Magnifies worries. Impedes emotional regulation and coping skills.

- Promotes weight gain and fat storage, especially unhealthy belly fat depositing around the abdomen.

- Induces insulin resistance and worsens blood sugar regulation, increasing diabetes risk.

- Aggravates skin conditions like acne, eczema and psoriasis. Accelerates visible signs of ageing.

- Disrupts hormonal balance including sex hormones and stress hormones. Can affect fertility and libido.

- Impacts cellular ageing by shortening telomeres, the protective sequences at the end of chromosomes.

- Worsens pain perception and aggravates chronic pain conditions. Amplifies physical discomfort.

- Contributes to headaches and migraines. Causes muscle tension, spasms and discomfort.

- Impairs sleep quality and leads to fatigue. Causes racing thoughts that interfere with rest.

Relaxation Techniques

Practising relaxation techniques activates the parasympathetic nervous system to counteract the stress response and induce calmness. Here are some approaches:

Deep Breathing: Taking slow, mindful breaths signals safety to the body which can lower blood pressure, heart rate, and anxiety levels. Breathe deeply into the abdomen rather than shallow chest breathing. Count to 4 on the inhale, pause, then count to

5-6 on the exhale. Repeat for several minutes.

Progressive Muscle Relaxation: Systematically tense and relax muscle groups throughout the body to release physical tension. Start with the toes, feet and lower leg, hold tension briefly, then relax. Repeat with thighs, back, stomach, arms, neck and face.

Guided Imagery: Use vivid mental images of calm, peaceful scenes to shift focus. Picture walking along the beach, through a forest, or other serene landscapes engaging all your senses. Allow thoughts to pass without judgement if your mind wanders.

Mindfulness Meditation: Focus intently on an anchor like your breath, a repeated word or object in your surroundings to ground yourself in the present moment rather than dwelling on worries. Acknowledge wandering thoughts then gently return focus to the anchor.

Breathing Exercises

In addition to deep, diaphragmatic breathing practice, specific breathing exercises can enhance relaxation:

- 4-7-8 Breathing: Inhale for 4 slow counts, hold breath for 7 counts, then exhale fully for 8 counts. Repeat for 4-5 breath cycles to reduce anxiety.

- Alternate Nostril Breathing: Gently close off one nostril while inhaling fully through the open nostril. Switch to exhale through the opposite nostril. Continue alternating nostrils for multiple breath cycles. Helps balance energy.

- Sitali Breathing: Curl your tongue lengthwise with the sides pressed against the teeth. Inhale slowly through the tongue then close your mouth and exhale normally through your nose. Aids in cooling and reduces agitation.

- Humming Bee Breath: Inhale through your nose then humm or buzz loudly on the exhale with lips gently closed, like the sound of a bee. Vibrations calm the nervous system.

Mindfulness and Meditation

Mindfulness and meditation practices strengthen concentration, emotion regulation, stress resilience, and overall well being:

- Mindfulness Meditation involves nonjudgmental awareness and acceptance of moment-to-moment experiences. Rather than worrying about the future or rehashing the past, mindful presence grounds you in the now. This releases perceived stressors that are out of your control. Apps like Headspace provide excellent guided sessions.

- Loving-Kindness Meditation focuses on self-acceptance and cultivating compassion for yourself and others by mentally offering positive intentions, wishes and forgiveness. Visualising offering and receiving kindness increases positive emotions and reduces hostility.

- Transcendental Meditation uses the silent repetition of a mantra or meaningful sound to achieve a tranquil, wakeful state of restful awareness. No concentration or control of the mind is required. Studies show decreased anxiety and blood pressure along with boosted mood after regular practice.

- Walking Meditation synergizes gentle physical movement with mindfulness of bodily sensations during a slow mindful walk. Feel the ground under your feet and sway of your limbs while staying focused on the present. Being in nature enhances benefits.

Yoga and Stretching

Yoga postures and stretching routines alleviate muscle tension and rebalance the nervous system:

- Yoga coordinates breathing with sequenced postures that build strength, flexibility, and mindfulness. Movement is synchronised with inhales and exhales. Studies confirm yoga lowers stress hormones, anxiety, inflammation and cardiovascular risk markers.

- Stretching elongates tense muscles and enhances body awareness. Rotate your head and shoulders, interlace your fingers to stretch arms overhead, extend your spine, and release your hips to reduce accumulated tension and rediscover ease of movement.

Lifestyle Adjustments

Along with specific relaxation techniques, making certain lifestyle modifications can significantly decrease stress:

- Set reasonable expectations for yourself and relinquish perfectionism. Avoid overcommitting. Learn to say no. Delegate or remove unnecessary obligations.

- Incorporate stress relievers into each day like relaxing baths, soothing music, enjoyable hobbies, reflecting in a journal, or time with supportive loved ones.

- Limit exposure to stressful news and media if it feels overwhelming. Seek positive content instead. Turn off screens and devices at a set time nightly.

- Make time for proper sleep, regular exercise, and nutritious food to strengthen your resiliency. Maintain balance between productivity and self-care.

- If a certain situation or relationship consistently causes distress, assess ways to improve it. If not possible, limiting contact may be warranted.

- Take mini-breaks throughout the day to move, stretch,

enjoy calming tea, briefly meditate or do light yoga poses. Even 2-3 minutes of relaxation refreshes.

- Spend time in nature as often as possible. Forest bathing, walking on the beach, hiking and other green activities restore inner calm.

- If work burnout, anxiety or depression make daily function difficult, seek counselling support and possible medication to regain equilibrium. Asking for help is brave.

Identifying Stress Triggers

Determining which situations tend to trigger your stress response allows conscious efforts toward avoidance or adaptation:

- Monitor your mood and write down circumstances, times of day, interactions, thoughts or environments associated with heightened tension.

- Look for patterns about whether stress centres around particular relationships, work pressures, pessimistic thought cycles, lack of self-care, limited downtime or not asserting boundaries.

- Once you identify key themes, brainstorm potential solutions. Perhaps increased social support, a new job, thought pattern adjustments, setting firmer boundaries or adding relaxing rituals to your schedule would help.

- While some stress triggers can be minimised, others may need to be accepted. Focus energy on modifying elements within your control. Let go of uncontrollable things.

- Be compassionate with yourself. Certain vulnerable times like holidays, anniversaries or milestones may require extra self-care and social support. The key is cultivating resilience.

Seeking Professional Help

For chronic, unremitting stress that persists despite your best efforts, seeking outside treatment is wise. A combination of therapy, medication, and lifestyle changes may be needed:

- Psychotherapy helps build coping skills, shift thought patterns, improve relationships and address underlying issues fuelling stress. Therapists impart tools tailored to your unique needs.

- Medications like certain antidepressants and anti-anxiety drugs can be prescribed for short-term use to restore calm, balance brain chemistry and manage debilitating symptoms in tandem with therapy.

- Psychiatrists can assess if medications are indicated to address anxiety, depression, insomnia or other issues aggravated by excess stress. Related conditions may need targeted treatment.

- Joining a support group provides encouragement, accountability and a sense you are not alone. Shared experiences build compassion and possibility.

- Developing a holistic self-care plan with a counsellor considering diet, exercise, socialisation, relaxation practices and nature exposure in addition to therapy and medication can maximise benefits.

In summary, a multi-pronged stress relief approach centred around self-care, lifestyle adjustments, therapeutic techniques, social support and professional help when warranted allows you to regain balance and cultivate resilience in the face of life's inevitable challenges. With compassion for yourself and others, peace and equanimity remain possible.

CHAPTER 5: SLEEPING YOUR WAY TO HEALTH

Sleep is profoundly important for overall health and wellbeing. However, many struggle with insufficient or poor-quality sleep due to ingrained habits, medical issues or modern lifestyles. Prioritising healthy sleep hygiene practices, establishing beneficial bedtime rituals, managing common sleep disorders through lifestyle changes and medical support when needed, and understanding when professional help should be sought all contribute to getting your best rest on a consistent basis.

The Importance of Sleep for Overall Health

Sleep allows the body and mind to restore, repair and recharge. Getting enough high-quality sleep is crucial:

- Supports immune function. Sleep deprivation increases susceptibility to sickness.

- Enhances learning, memory, focus and productivity. Allows brain connections to strengthen.

- Helps regulate metabolism, appetite and weight. Curbs

cravings and overeating.

- Lowers risk for chronic diseases like heart disease, diabetes and cancer.

- Reduces inflammation throughout the body that contributes to disease when unchecked.

- Balances mood and emotional reactivity. Lessens anxiety and depression.

- Normalizes blood pressure and cardiovascular function. Protects heart health.

- Allows muscles and tissues to heal and renew. Promotes growth and development.

- Removes toxic cellular byproducts accumulated during waking hours. Detoxifies.

- Boosters sex hormone production. Important for fertility and libido.

Signs of Poor Sleep Quality

Indicators that sleep quality or duration may be suboptimal:

- Frequent insomnia or difficulty falling/staying asleep

- Reliance on sleeping pills or alcohol to sleep

- Waking up feeling unrefreshed. Ongoing fatigue or sleepiness during the day.

- Difficulty focusing, learning new things, remembering details

- Increased irritability, mood swings, anxiety or signs of depression

- Ongoing muscle tension, headaches or gastrointestinal issues

- Hypertension or increased resting heart rate

- Increased hunger, cravings or unintentional weight gain

- Lower immunity with frequent colds

If poor sleep persists for weeks, it likely signifies an issue needing attention.

Tips for Improving Sleep Hygiene

Sleep hygiene refers to conditions, habits and practices that promote consistent, high-quality sleep. Good sleep hygiene:

- Maintain a consistent sleep schedule, even on weekends. Aim for 7-9 hours nightly for adults.

- Establish relaxing pre-bedtime routines like reading, gentle yoga or taking a bath.

- Avoid electronic devices and screens for 1-2 hours before bedtime. The blue light interferes with circadian rhythms.

- Make the bedroom cool, completely dark and quiet. Consider blackout curtains, a white noise machine or ear plugs.

- Choose a comfortable mattress and pillow that allows spinal alignment. Replace regularly.

- Avoid large meals, caffeine or alcohol before bed, which can disrupt sleep. Finish eating 2-3 hours before bedtime.

- Limit daytime napping to 30 minutes or less. Try to nap before 3 pm to avoid interfering with nighttime sleep.

- Move your body and get exposure to daylight during the day to help regulate circadian rhythms.

- If you don't fall asleep within 20 minutes or wake up and can't fall back asleep within 20 minutes, get out of bed and try a relaxing activity until drowsy.

Establishing Beneficial Bedtime Habits and Rituals

Incorporating consistent relaxing rituals into the hour before bed makes it easier to unwind and transition into quality sleep:

- Take a warm bath or shower to relax muscles and induce drowsiness. Add epsom salts or lavender oil.

- Sip chamomile or other herbal tea to promote relaxation.

- Practise deep breathing exercises to reduce racing thoughts and quiet the mind.

- Do gentle, restorative yoga poses to release stored muscle tension.

- Write thoughts and to-do lists on paper to clear your mind for sleep.

- Play soft, calming music like nature sounds or classical to wind down.

- Diffuse calming essential oils like lavender or eucalyptus to create a soothing environment.

- Turn down the thermostat slightly. Cooler room temperatures enhance sleep.

- Read an uplifting book that doesn't provoke anxiety or stimulate brain activity.

- Try mindfulness or light meditation to detach from worries and be present.

Managing Common Sleep Difficulties and Disorders

Lifestyle adjustments, natural remedies and medical treatment can help manage sleep obstacles:

Insomnia: Difficulty falling or staying asleep.

- Establish a relaxing pre-bed routine and sleep

environment

- Avoid screens before bed

- Try natural remedies like chamomile tea, magnesium supplements or CBD oil

- Talk to your doctor about short-term sleep aid medication if needed

- Consider Cognitive Behavioral Therapy (CBT) techniques to change sleep thoughts and habits

Restless Leg Syndrome: Uncomfortable leg sensations that disrupt sleep.

- Reduce caffeine and do moderate exercise during the day

- Take warm baths, do leg stretches or massage before bed

- Discuss supplementing with magnesium, iron or folate with your doctor

- Prescription medications like dopamine agonists, benzodiazepines or opioids may be options

Sleep Apnea: Repeated pauses in breathing during sleep.

- Practise proper sleep position by sleeping on your side instead of back

- Maintain healthy body weight and physical fitness

- Avoid alcohol and sedatives

- A CPAP machine prescribed by a doctor helps maintain airflow

Delayed Sleep Phase Disorder: Extreme night owl pattern and difficulty waking in the mornings.

- Use light therapy in the mornings to reset circadian rhythm

- Take melatonin several hours before target bedtime

- Stick to a fixed sleep schedule, even on weekends

- Seek counselling if underlying emotional issues or depression are present

When to Seek Professional Help

If poor sleep persists despite practising good sleep hygiene for 3-4 weeks or severely impairs function, seek medical advice:

- A primary care doctor can check for underlying conditions like chronic pain, gastrointestinal reflux, hyperthyroidism or depression contributing to sleep problems. Bloodwork might identify deficiencies.

- Sleep specialists can conduct thorough assessments, recommend sleep studies to diagnose issues like sleep apnea, and provide customised treatment plans.

- Cognitive behavioural therapy for insomnia from a licensed psychologist or counsellor can help unlearn harmful thought patterns and behaviours around sleep.

- Sleep clinics offer comprehensive evaluations and access to specialists who collaborate to restore healthy sleep.

- A psychiatrist can prescribe sleep medications or treat psychiatric disorders like anxiety, PTSD or bipolar disorder that affect sleep.

- Alternative practitioners like naturopaths, acupuncturists or massage therapists may complement medical treatment with natural remedies, herbs, essential oils, meditation, etc. For overall well being.

- Support groups connect you with others struggling with sleep disorders. Shared understanding boosts motivation.

In summary, prioritising healthy sleep is one of the best things you can do for your overall health and longevity. Start with good sleep hygiene basics, establish calming bedtime routines, address any sleep issues through lifestyle changes and medical support, and seek professional treatment when needed. With commitment, healthy, restorative sleep is within your reach.

CHAPTER 6: EMBRACING NATURE'S REMEDIES

Harnessing the healing properties of nutritious foods, beneficial herbs and supplements allows you to take an active role in supporting health and wellbeing. However, natural remedies may interact with medications or medical conditions, so working with healthcare providers and using caution is essential. When approached responsibly, nature offers accessible and effective solutions.

Using Foods as Natural Medicine

Certain foods contain powerful compounds that prevent or treat various ailments. Incorporating them into meals provides therapeutic benefits:

Inflammation: Chronic inflammation contributes to nearly all major diseases. Choose foods high in anti-inflammatory compounds:

- Omega-3 fatty acids: Found in oily fish, walnuts, flax and chia seeds. Help treat arthritis, autoimmune disorders, heart disease and dementia.

- Anthocyanins: Found in berries, red grapes, red cabbage and dark greens. Protect cardiovascular health and brain function.

- Sulforaphane: Found in cruciferous vegetables like broccoli, kale and Brussels sprouts. May help prevent cancer.

- Curcumin: Found in turmeric spice. Used as anti-inflammatory for arthritis and autoimmunity.

- Quercetin: Found in apples, onions and tea. Used to reduce allergy symptoms and pain.

High Blood Pressure: Also called hypertension, high blood pressure strains arteries and endangers heart health. Eat more:

- Bananas: Rich in potassium, which regulates fluid balance and reduces pressure on blood vessel walls.

- Beetroot: Nitrates in beets dilate blood vessels and improve blood flow.

- Oats: Soluble fibre in oats binds to cholesterol to lower blood pressure.

- Flaxseeds: Provide magnesium, potassium and fibre for pressure reduction.

- Garlic: Helps expand blood vessels. Can also be taken as a supplement.

High Blood Sugar: Uncontrolled elevated blood sugar can lead to prediabetes and type 2 diabetes. Choose foods that help regulate blood sugar by slowing digestion and insulin release:

- Whole grains like oats, quinoa, brown rice and buckwheat.

- Legumes including beans, peas and lentils which are rich in fibre and protein.

- Nuts such as almonds, walnuts and peanuts contain healthy fats, fibre and protein.

- Berries are packed with antioxidants and fibre to slow sugar absorption.

- Leafy greens like spinach help manage blood glucose levels.

Immunity: Booster immune defences against pathogens naturally with these foods:

- Citrus fruits high in vitamin C like oranges, grapefruit and clementines.

- Shiitake, maitake and oyster mushrooms have antiviral and infection-fighting properties.

- Yogurt and kefir provide probiotics to balance gut bacteria and strengthen immunity.

- Garlic possesses antimicrobial, antibacterial and antifungal properties.

- Ginger is anti-inflammatory and contains antimicrobial compounds like gingerol.

Herbal Remedies and Precautions

Traditional herbal remedies can be beneficial when used appropriately:

Echinacea: Boosts immune function and combats colds. Often taken as a tincture or tea. Avoid long-term use.

Elderberry: Provides antioxidants that relieve cold/flu symptoms. Available as syrups, gummies or teas. May interact with autoimmune medications.

Turmeric/Curcumin: Has anti-inflammatory effects that help treat arthritis when taken in supplement form. Do not consume medicinal doses without physician oversight.

Valerian Root: Promotes sleep and reduces anxiety. Use caution with sedative medications or liver issues. Best taken temporarily.

Chamomile Tea: Soothes upset stomach, relieves anxiety and aids sleep. Avoid pregnancy. Rarely causes allergic reaction.

Ginger: Settles nausea and digestive issues. Effective for morning sickness but check with your doctor during pregnancy. Moderation recommended.

Ginkgo Biloba: Taken for memory enhancement but clinical results are mixed. Has blood thinning effects. Use caution with clotting disorders.

Saw Palmetto: Used for benign prostatic hyperplasia (BPH) in men but evidence is limited. Avoid during pregnancy or with hormone-sensitive cancers.

As with any supplement, inform your healthcare provider about any herbal remedies you take to prevent interactions with medications or health conditions. Only use reputable brands and follow dosing guidelines.

Benefits and Risks of Nutritional Supplements

Dietary supplements can offer advantages when used strategically but also have associated risks:

Potential Benefits

- Multivitamins help fill nutrition gaps and promote wellness, especially during high stress times, pregnancy or if deficiencies are present.

- Vitamin D, magnesium and calcium support bone health and prevent osteoporosis when sufficient dietary intake is difficult.

- Omega-3 fish oil supplements provide anti-inflammatory and heart health benefits, especially for those who dislike fish.

- Probiotics aid digestion and immunity by enhancing populations of beneficial bacteria, particularly after illness or antibiotics.

- Protein powders offer supplemental protein for building muscle, especially for athletes, seniors or those recovering from surgery.

- Melatonin, taken short-term, can help reset sleep cycles for those having trouble with sleep onset or jet lag recovery.

Potential Risks

- Very high doses of some vitamins like A, D, E, iron and calcium can be harmful. Stick to recommended daily values.

- Safety standards for supplement manufacturing are not as stringent as prescription drugs, so quality issues are sometimes a concern.

- Some herbal supplements like St. John's Wort negatively interact with medications. Knowing interactions is essential.

- Over-supplementing in lieu of a balanced diet provides an excess of isolated nutrients that might do more harm than good.

- Individuals with pre-existing conditions need physician guidance, as supplements can complicate some diseases if taken inappropriately.

For optimal safety and effectiveness, take supplements only after addressing dietary gaps and consult your doctor to confirm they are appropriate for your needs and health status. Moderation and care are key.

Popular Natural Treatments for Common Ailments

Natural remedies using foods, herbs and supplements may help treat minor ailments:

Stomach upset: Ginger, chamomile or peppermint tea, fennel, BRAT diet (bananas, rice, applesauce, toast)

Minor cuts and scrapes: Turmeric, tea tree oil, raw honey

Seasonal allergies: Local honey, quercetin, stinging nettle, vitamin C

Cold sores: Lysine supplements, lemon balm, licorice root cream

Mild anxiety: Chamomile, passionflower, valerian root, magnesium, yoga

Headaches: Peppermint essential oil, feverfew, magnesium, BCAA supplements

Trouble sleeping: Glycine, melatonin, valerian root, magnesium, chamomile tea

Indigestion/heartburn: DGL licorice, slippery elm, marshmallow root, ginger tea

Muscle cramps and soreness: Magnesium, potassium, Arnica gel, gentle stretching

For relief of chronic issues or moderate to severe symptoms, consult your physician about effective medical treatment. Do not attempt to self-treat serious conditions without professional advice.

Potential Interactions with Medications

Some foods, herbs and supplements can interact with over-the-counter or prescription medications through various mechanisms:

- Blood thinner interactions: Vitamin E, fish oil, gingko, turmeric/curcumin, ginger and garlic can increase bleeding risks when taken alongside blood-thinning medications like warfarin or aspirin.

- Absorption interference: Calcium may inhibit absorption of thyroid medications while high-fibre foods reduce absorption of some antibiotics if taken at the same time.

- Medication breakdown: The liver breaks down substances via the cytochrome P450 pathway. Herbs like St. John's Wort induce these enzymes which can speed up breakdown of medications, reducing effectiveness.

- Drug interactions: Mixing stimulants found in some herbs and supplements with drugs that have similar effects like increasing blood pressure or heart rate could compound the effects.

Always inform your doctor about any herbs, supplements or functional foods you take so the potential for any interactions can be reviewed. Reputable brands will caution about known medication interactions on their labels. When in doubt, professional guidance is key.

Working With Healthcare Providers

Navigating natural remedies calls for open collaboration with your doctor:

- Share any herbs, supplements or functional foods you take, their dose, frequency, and the intended purpose. This allows assessment for possible medication interactions.

- Consult your doctor before beginning any new herbal remedy, particularly if you have a chronic health condition, take prescription medications, or are pregnant/ breastfeeding. Professional oversight helps minimise risks.

- Ask your doctor for reliable supplement brands they recommend and dosage guidelines to ensure safety and efficacy. Following practitioner advice is key.

- Be skeptical of claims herbal products can "cure" complex conditions. Your doctor can provide an evidence-based perspective on validity and possible benefits.

- For a holistic approach, consult naturopathic doctors or professionals trained in integrative medicine to safely combine conventional and natural treatments.

- Nutritionists can help you formulate a diet using functional foods to prevent or manage health conditions. A balanced approach is ideal.

Partnering with healthcare providers to make informed decisions ensures natural remedies enhance your wellness safely and strategically. While nature provides us with healing foods and herbs, professional guidance maximises their benefits while avoiding potential pitfalls.

CHAPTER 7: PREVENTING AND MANAGING CHRONIC DISEASE

Chronic diseases like heart disease, diabetes, cancer, and Alzheimer's represent the leading causes of disability and death worldwide. However, research confirms that lifestyle factors like diet, exercise, sleep and stress management significantly influence chronic disease risk. Making proactive changes along with working closely with healthcare providers allows you to take control of your health.

The Role of Lifestyle in Chronic Disease Risk

While genetics and non-modifiable factors like age and family history play a part, research reveals that poor lifestyle habits contribute to up to 80% of chronic disease cases. Key risk factors include:

- Physical inactivity and sedentary behaviours like excessive sitting

- Obesity and carrying excess body fat, especially visceral

abdominal fat

- Unhealthy dietary patterns high in processed foods, added sugars, refined carbs, and inflammatory fats

- Smoking or excessive alcohol intake

- Chronic stress, anxiety, and inadequate sleep

- Exposure to environmental pollutants and toxins

- Lack of meaningful social connections and community support

Conversely, those who engage in healthy lifestyle practices like regular exercise, whole food diets, stress management, restorative sleep, and social involvement slash chronic disease risks significantly.

Diet and Exercise Recommendations for Prevention

Research-backed diet and exercise guidelines help reduce chances of developing major chronic illnesses:

Heart Disease and Stroke

- Follow a heart-healthy diet like the Mediterranean diet emphasising vegetables, fruits, whole grains, legumes, nuts, fish and olive oil. Limit red meat and sweets.

- Engage in 150 minutes per week of moderate exercise like brisk walking or 75 minutes weekly of vigorous exercise like running.

- Strength train 2-3 times per week to improve lean muscle mass, bone density and cardiovascular health markers.

- Achieve and maintain a lean BMI through calorie management and daily activity. Carrying excess weight strains the heart.

Diabetes

- Choose minimally processed, low glycemic index foods like non-starchy vegetables, legumes, nuts, whole grains, and lean proteins to maintain steady blood sugar.

- Exercise helps improve insulin sensitivity and keep blood sugar balanced. Both aerobic and strength training are beneficial.

- Work towards a healthy body weight since excess body fat, especially around the abdomen, contributes to diabetes risk. Losing just 5-10% of weight helps.

- If diabetic, diligent glucose testing, insulin administration as prescribed, routine medical oversight, and prompt treatment of related conditions like high cholesterol or nerve damage are essential.

Cancer

- Emphasise a diet rich in fruits, vegetables, whole grains and lean proteins. Phytochemicals, fibre, vitamins and minerals in plant foods help protect cells.

- Engage in at least 150 minutes weekly of moderate activity which helps circulation and reduces inflammation. Physical activity is associated with lower cancer incidence.

- Reach and preserve a healthy BMI through balanced nutrition and routine exercise. Obesity increases risk for at least 13 different cancers.

- Avoid tobacco and excess alcohol which are carcinogenic and mutagenic chemicals that directly damage DNA leading to cancer initiation and growth.

Alzheimer's and Dementia

- Follow a Mediterranean style diet which emphasises produce, whole grains, olive oil and fish for optimal brain nutrition and blood flow. The MIND diet adds nuts and berries.

- Aerobic exercise several times weekly boosts blood flow to the brain and releases growth factors like brain-derived neurotrophic factors that support brain cell health.

- Mental stimulation through learning new skills, reading, puzzles and social activities forms cognitive reserve that maintain neuron connections to delay onset of Alzheimer's symptoms.

- Manage stress levels and prioritise 7+ hours of sleep nightly. Chronic stress and poor sleep are linked to cognitive decline and dementia development.

Other Preventive Measures

- Avoid smoking and secondhand smoke exposure which harms nearly every organ system. Get support in the quitting process.

- Limit alcohol consumption to 1 drink daily for women or 2 for men at most. Heavy alcohol use damages the liver, heart and nervous system.

- Minimise exposure to air pollution and environmental toxins which promote inflammation and free radical damage. Use appropriate safety equipment if exposures are occupational.

- Adopt stress relieving practices like mindfulness, social connection, yoga, nature exposure and adequate sleep to counter the effects of chronic stress. If needed, seek counselling support.

- Take advantage of preventive health services like cancer screenings, routine check-ups, and vaccinations. Early detection of conditions allows earlier intervention.

Managing Existing Illnesses Through Lifestyle

Even after being diagnosed with chronic diseases, lifestyle still matters:

Heart Disease

- Closely adhere to prescribed heart medications, regular monitoring and any dietary/activity recommendations from your cardiologist. Carry emergency medications like nitroglycerin if applicable.

- Follow a heart-healthy diet focusing on produce, whole grains, lean protein and healthy fats while limiting sodium, sugar and unhealthy fats. Drink adequate water.

- Do regular moderate physical activity aiming for 30 minutes daily. However, check with your doctor for personalised exercise guidelines based on disease severity.

- Lose excess weight if overweight. Avoid smoking. Manage stress levels through healthy outlets and maintain relationships. Join a cardiac rehab program if applicable.

Diabetes

- Monitor blood glucose routinely through finger prick tests or a continuous glucose monitor. Track results and share them with your care team.

- Take medications or insulin as prescribed and learn how to balance medication, food and activity to keep blood sugar controlled.

- Follow a diabetic diet emphasising complex carbohydrates, fibre and lean proteins while limiting simple sugars, refined grains and unhealthy fats. Portion control is key.

- Incorporate both aerobic and resistance exercise to improve insulin sensitivity and maintain muscle mass, following exercise guidelines from your diabetic care team.

- Use proper foot care, dental hygiene, skin protection and seek treatment for related issues like neuropathy or eye disease to avoid diabetes complications. Get routine medical oversight.

Cancer

- Follow specialised dietary guidelines from your oncologist during treatment. Supportive nutrition helps you maintain strength, energy and resilience.

- Do light activity regularly within limits set by your physician. Even short walks can reduce treatment side effects and fatigue.

- Integrative approaches like acupuncture, massage and mindfulness may complement conventional treatment by reducing stress and pain. Consult your care team.

- Join a support group to share your cancer journey with others who understand. Social support eases isolation and hopelessness.

- Examine lifestyle habits like diet and activity levels post-treatment to make positive changes that promote recovery and lower recurrence risks.

Alzheimer's and Dementia

- Work closely with your care team regarding medications to slow progression, managing behaviour changes, home safety strategies, social support and outpacing care needs as cognition declines. Take meds as directed.

- Maintain nutritious and routine meals with simple preparation. Focus on easily chewed whole foods and hydration. Supplements can fill nutrition gaps.

- Do regular light exercise like walking outdoors when possible for physical and emotional benefits. Discontinue exercise immediately if it causes distress.

- Engage in memory games, puzzles, reminiscing and recreational activities that provide cognitive stimulation and social connection within ability level. Music, art, and pets can enrich life.

- Modify communication approaches like using visual cues, keeping instructions simple, repetition, and reassuring touches to sustain relationships despite cognitive impairment.

Working with Healthcare Providers

Prevention and management of chronic diseases requires active partnership with providers:

- See your doctor for routine visits, health screenings like mammography or colonoscopy, needed vaccinations, prompt work ups for unusual symptoms and management of existing diseases.

- Create a collaborative relationship with providers. Share your lifestyle, priorities and desired level of involvement in your care. Ask questions if anything is unclear.

- Register with the patient portal through your health system. Portal messaging, appointment scheduling and access to test results promotes efficiency.

- Make medication adherence, regular lab tests, and other provider recommendations a priority. Complete needed follow up rest ordered. Preventive health cannot be neglected.

- Discuss any proposed lifestyle changes, supplements or natural remedies with your physician to ensure safety and appropriateness considering your medical status and prescribed medications which could interact.

- For severe or complex conditions, partnering with a health-focused care coordinator at your medical centre facilitates navigation of multi-disciplinary medical care.

The Importance of Early Detection

Detecting chronic illnesses early substantially improves prognosis and survival rates:

- Routine recommended health screenings allow diseases like breast, cervical, colorectal and prostate cancers to be caught at preliminary stages when they are most treatable.

- Lab tests during annual physicals can uncover issues like high cholesterol, blood sugar or calcium levels before they progress to overt heart disease, diabetes or osteoporosis.

- Seeking medical attention promptly for concerning symptoms reduces chances a minor condition will escalate. Symptoms like change in bowel habits, unexplained bleeding or weight loss, headaches, chest pain, or breathing issues should never be ignored.

- Making use of patient portals for test results allows you to view and track changes in health metrics. Early intervention may be prompted before deterioration is clinically obvious.

- Genetic testing helps identify inherited predispositions to certain cancers and other diseases. Knowing individual risks allows tailored prevention and surveillance steps.

In summary, fostering daily healthy habits, developing

awareness of changes in your body, undergoing recommended screening examinations, adhering to regular medical care including tests and vaccinations, and addressing issues early is the recipe for successfully avoiding or overcoming chronic illness. Your health trajectory is far from fixed. Commit to prevention and early action for your best life!

CHAPTER 8:
HEALTHY LIVING
FOR LONGEVITY

Embarking on a journey towards healthy living is a commitment to prioritise well-being, vitality, and longevity. This comprehensive guide explores various facets of cultivating a healthy lifestyle, emphasising the importance of making gradual changes, sustaining new habits, continuous education, collaboration with professionals, and recognising wellness as a lifelong endeavour. By understanding the benefits of healthy living, individuals can take proactive steps towards not only extending their lifespan but also enhancing their overall quality of life.

Before delving into the specifics of healthy living, let's take a moment to review the key areas we'll be exploring:

1. Making Changes Gradually: The significance of adopting a phased approach to lifestyle modifications for sustainable and lasting results.

2. Sticking with New Healthy Habits: Strategies for reinforcing and maintaining positive changes in daily routines.

3. Ongoing Education: The role of continuous learning in staying informed about the latest health trends and evidence-based practices.

4. Working with Professionals: The importance of seeking guidance from healthcare providers, nutritionists, and fitness experts.

5. Wellness as a Lifelong Journey: Recognizing that well-being is a dynamic, lifelong process that evolves over time.

6. Benefits of Healthy Living for Longevity: Understanding how a healthy lifestyle contributes to a longer, more fulfilling life.

Making Changes Gradually

The Power of Incremental Progress

1. Setting Realistic Goals: Establishing achievable objectives lays the foundation for long-term success.

2. Prioritising Consistency: Gradual changes that become consistent habits are more likely to endure.

3. Focusing on Small Adjustments: Incremental shifts in behaviour are easier to integrate and sustain.

4. Building a Support System: Surrounding oneself with a supportive community can reinforce commitment to change.

5. Embracing Patience: Recognizing that lasting transformation takes time fosters a positive mindset.

Sticking with New Healthy Habits

Strategies for Sustained Well-being

1. Creating a Routine: Establishing a structured daily schedule reinforces healthy habits.

2. Monitoring Progress: Tracking improvements provides motivation and reinforces commitment.

3. Celebrating Milestones: Acknowledging achievements, no matter how small, reinforces positive behaviour.

4. Adapting to Challenges: Responding flexibly to setbacks fosters resilience and prevents discouragement.

5. Practising Mindfulness: Being present in the moment enhances self-awareness and reinforces healthy choices.

Ongoing Education

The Quest for Knowledge and Growth

1. Staying Informed: Regularly seeking out credible sources of health information ensures up-to-date knowledge.

2. Exploring Diverse Perspectives: Gaining insights from a variety of sources broadens one's understanding of well-being.

3. Attending Workshops and Seminars: Participating in educational events fosters continuous learning.

4. Reading Health Literature: Books, articles, and research papers are valuable resources for deepening knowledge.

5. Engaging in Online Communities: Joining forums or social media groups focused on health provides opportunities for learning and sharing experiences.

Working with Professionals

Leveraging Expertise for Optimal Health

1. Regular Health Check-ups: Scheduling routine appointments with healthcare providers allows for early detection and prevention.

2. Consulting Nutritionists: Seeking advice from qualified nutritionists ensures balanced and nourishing dietary choices.

3. Engaging Fitness Experts: Working with certified fitness trainers ensures safe and effective exercise routines.

4. Collaborating with Mental Health Professionals: Seeking therapy or counselling supports emotional well-being and resilience.

5. Exploring Alternative Therapies: Integrating practices like acupuncture, chiropractic care, or massage therapy can complement conventional treatments.

Wellness as a Lifelong Journey

Embracing the Continuum of Well-being

1. Adapting to Life Changes: Recognizing that wellness needs may shift over time allows for necessary adjustments.

2. Embracing Ageing Gracefully: Understanding that well-being is not static empowers individuals to navigate the natural ageing process.

3. Prioritising Self-Care: Consistently making time for self-care activities fosters ongoing physical and mental health.

4. Cultivating Resilience: Building emotional and physical resilience supports long-term well-being.

5. Nurturing Relationships: Meaningful connections contribute significantly to overall life satisfaction and well-being.

Benefits of Healthy Living for Longevity

The Rewards of Prioritising Well-being

1. Extended Lifespan: Scientific research consistently demonstrates that a healthy lifestyle can lead to a longer life.

2. Enhanced Quality of Life: Well-being is not only about length of life but also about the richness and fulfilment experienced throughout it.

3. Reduced Risk of Chronic Diseases: Healthy living significantly lowers the likelihood of developing common chronic conditions like heart disease, diabetes, and hypertension.

4. Optimised Cognitive Function: A balanced lifestyle supports cognitive health, reducing the risk of cognitive decline and disorders like dementia.

5. Improved Emotional Well-being: Physical health and emotional well-being are intricately linked, and a healthy lifestyle contributes to positive mental health outcomes.

Conclusion

Healthy living for longevity is a multifaceted endeavour that encompasses a holistic approach to well-being. By embracing gradual changes, sustaining new habits, pursuing ongoing education, collaborating with professionals, and recognizing wellness as a lifelong journey, individuals can unlock the full potential of their health. Understanding the myriad benefits of healthy living not only extends one's lifespan but also enhances overall quality of life. Through this comprehensive guide, individuals are empowered to embark on a journey towards a longer, more vibrant, and fulfilling existence.

CHAPTER 9: COCONUT OIL AND ANTIMICROBIAL PROPERTIES: A CLOSER LOOK

Coconut oil has received a lot of attention in recent years as a potential antimicrobial agent. Here, we take a closer look at the current scientific evidence regarding coconut oil and its antimicrobial properties.

What are antimicrobials?

Antimicrobials are substances that kill or inhibit the growth of microorganisms like bacteria, fungi, parasites and viruses. Antimicrobial agents play an important role in fighting infectious diseases and preventing the spread of pathogens.

Does coconut oil have antimicrobial properties?

Coconut oil contains several fatty acids that have been shown to have antimicrobial effects, particularly lauric acid. In studies, lauric acid demonstrated antibacterial, antifungal and antiviral properties. Other coconut oil components like capric acid and caprylic acid also exhibited some antimicrobial activities.

How does lauric acid in coconut oil act as an antimicrobial?

Lauric acid is converted into a substance called monolaurin in the body. Both lauric acid and monolaurin can disrupt lipid membranes and interfere with critical microbial functions, leading to cell disintegration and death. This effect is more pronounced on lipid-coated viruses, bacteria and yeasts.

What does the research say?

Studies have shown coconut oil and its components like lauric acid inhibited the growth of specific bacteria like Streptococcus mutans, Staphylococcus aureus and Helicobacter pylori. It has also demonstrated antifungal effects against Candida species. However, the research is limited and most studies used concentrations much higher than typical dietary intake.

Are there any risks or downsides?

While coconut oil appears to have some antimicrobial properties, current evidence does not justify using it in place of prescribed antibiotics or antifungals. Self-medicating with coconut oil could also lead to allergic reactions or unanticipated side effects in some individuals.

Can it help fight infections?

There is insufficient evidence to recommend using coconut oil as a substitute for pharmaceutical drugs in treating infections. Coconut oil should not be solely relied upon to cure any illnesses without medical supervision. More research is still needed to determine safe and effective dosages.

The bottom line

Coconut oil does demonstrate potential antimicrobial properties, but the strength and clinical relevance of these effects remain to be fully established through large-scale human trials. Coconut oil should not replace conventional medical treatments proven to fight infections. More research is needed to develop any coconut oil-based antimicrobial therapies.

CHAPTER 10: THE POTENTIAL BENEFITS AND RISKS OF INTERMITTENT FASTING

Intermittent fasting has surged in popularity as a weight loss strategy in recent years. However, like most dietary approaches, it has both potential benefits and risks. Here, we review some of the science behind intermittent fasting.

What is intermittent fasting?

Intermittent fasting involves alternating between periods of fasting and eating. It does not specify which foods to eat, just when you should eat them. Common approaches include fasting for 16-48 hours 1-3 times per week or fasting for 12-16 hours daily.

Potential Benefits Of Intermittent Fasting:

- Weight loss: By limiting total calorie intake, intermittent fasting can lead to reduced body weight and body fat. However, results vary by individual.

- Lower blood pressure: Some studies have found intermittent fasting may reduce blood pressure, improving heart health. Effects seem more pronounced in those with elevated blood pressure.

- Improved blood sugar control: Intermittent fasting aids blood sugar regulation, which could benefit those with type 2 diabetes. However, more research is needed.

- Anti-ageing effects: Intermittent fasting may slow ageing processes by triggering autophagy and reducing oxidative stress and inflammation. However, human data is limited.

Potential Risks Of Intermittent Fasting:

- Nutrient deficiencies: Fasting periods restrict nutrient intake, which could lead to deficiencies over time. This depends on the overall diet.

- Dehydration: Longer fasts may increase dehydration risk if fluid intake is not increased during eating periods.

- Hunger and cravings: Intermittent fasting sometimes increases hunger, causing people to overeat during eating periods. This can undermine weight loss.

- Unrealistic long-term: Intermittent fasting is difficult to sustain forever. People may struggle to re-introduce regular eating habits post-fasting.

- Not for everyone: Intermittent fasting may be dangerous for those with a history of eating disorders or diabetes complications. Professional supervision is recommended.

The bottom line

When practised judiciously, intermittent fasting may provide some benefits such as weight loss. However, it does come with risks. It is critical to listen to your body's cues and stay hydrated. Consult a doctor before attempting intermittent fasting if you have any health conditions. Moderation and medically-supervised plans are recommended.

CHAPTER 11: APPLE CIDER VINEGAR

A Closer Look at the Potential Benefits and Risks of Apple Cider Vinegar

Apple cider vinegar has long been used as a folk remedy to treat a variety of health issues. In recent years, it has also gained popularity as a weight loss aid and "cure-all" tonic. But what does the science say about apple cider vinegar's purported benefits and risks? Here we take a closer look.

Potential Benefits

- Weight loss: Some small studies suggest vinegar may increase feelings of fullness after meals, which can support weight loss efforts. However, results are mixed.

- Blood sugar control: Vinegar may improve insulin sensitivity and blood sugar regulation, especially for those with insulin resistance or type 2 diabetes. However, human research is limited.

- Heart health: Some studies link vinegar consumption to improvements in blood pressure, cholesterol levels, and triglycerides. However, the evidence remains inconclusive.

- Antimicrobial effects: Laboratory tests indicate vinegar may inhibit the growth of some bacteria and viruses. However, human trials are needed.

Potential Risks

- Tooth enamel erosion: Vinegar's high acidity can degrade tooth enamel with regular consumption. Diluting it and avoiding swishing it around the mouth mitigates this risk.

- Digestive irritation: Apple cider vinegar may worsen conditions like heartburn or ulcers in those with gastrointestinal issues. It may also delay stomach emptying.

- Medication interactions: Theoretically, vinegar may interact with certain medications like insulin, diuretics, laxatives, and digoxin. Those on medications should consult a doctor before using it.

- Burn risk: Undiluted vinegar is highly acidic and can damage tissues if applied directly. Always dilute vinegar and avoid applying it directly to the skin and sensitive areas.

Bottom Line

Overall, the health benefits attributed to apple cider vinegar require more rigorous human research to confirm. While it displays some promise, its effects are often overstated. Vinegar consumption appears relatively safe for most people when used in moderation. However, it is critical to dilute it properly and avoid excessive intake to minimise potential risks. Those with certain medical conditions or on medications should exercise particular caution.

CHAPTER 12: AN ANALYSIS OF THE POTENTIAL HEALTH BENEFITS OF TURMERIC

Turmeric is a popular Indian spice that has been used for centuries in cooking and traditional medicine. In recent years, it has attracted attention due to its purported medicinal properties. Does science support the health claims about turmeric? Let's analyse the evidence.

What gives turmeric its potential benefits?

The active compound in turmeric is curcumin, which has demonstrated anti-inflammatory, antioxidant, and antimicrobial effects in lab studies. Curcumin may be responsible for many of turmeric's supposed therapeutic properties.

What does the research say about turmeric's benefits?

- Arthritis: Several studies show promise for

turmeric's ability to reduce joint inflammation and pain in osteoarthritis. The effects appear comparable to some anti-inflammatory drugs.

- Heart health: Curcumin may help improve blood flow and endothelial function. Turmeric's anti-inflammatory effects may also benefit those at risk of cardiovascular disease. But human data is limited.

- Cancer: Laboratory and animal studies indicate curcumin may stall cancer progression and development. However, clinical trials in humans are lacking.

- Cognition: Early studies suggest curcumin may boost cognition and mood in older adults. However, results are preliminary. Larger controlled studies are needed.

- Immunity: Turmeric exhibits antimicrobial properties in the lab. But there is insufficient clinical evidence showing it boosts immunity or treats infections.

Potential Risks And Considerations

At culinary doses, turmeric is considered very safe with minimal side effects. But medicinal doses may interact with some medications such as blood thinners and drugs affecting liver enzymes. There are also concerns about potential lead contamination in some turmeric supplements and powders. Always consult a doctor before using turmeric therapeutically, especially at high doses.

The bottom line

Overall, turmeric shows promise for certain conditions, but human data is limited. While low doses appear safe for most people, assumptions about therapeutic benefits should be tempered until larger clinical trials are conducted. Turmeric may be a helpful supplemental treatment, but it should not replace standard medical care.

CHAPTER 13: AN OBJECTIVE LOOK AT THE HEALTH EFFECTS OF DAIRY

Dairy products like milk, cheese, and yogurt are controversial when it comes to their health effects. While some view dairy as beneficial, others argue it may be inflammatory and harmful. What does science say about the pros and cons of dairy? Here, we review the evidence objectively.

Potential benefits of dairy consumption:

- Excellent source of calcium, vitamin D, and protein to support bone health

- Probiotics in yogurt can benefit digestive health

- Linked to lower blood pressure and reduced risk of cardiovascular disease

- Associated with decreased risk of type 2 diabetes

Potential Risks And Drawbacks Of Dairy

Consumption:

- Often high in saturated fat, which may negatively impact heart health

- Many people are intolerant or allergic to milk proteins (lactose intolerance, casein allergy)

- Possible increased risk of certain cancers (prostate, ovarian)

- Concerns about hormones and antibiotics found in conventional dairy

Effect Of Dairy On Inflammation:

- Dairy may trigger inflammation in those with milk allergies or sensitivities

- Fermented dairy like yogurt appears anti-inflammatory for most people

- Unprocessed dairy is likely neutral for those without intolerances

The bottom line

For people who tolerate it well, dairy can be a nutritious addition to an overall healthy diet, providing protein, vitamins, and minerals. However, whole milk dairy products should be consumed in moderation due to their saturated fat content. Individuals with sensitivities may need to avoid dairy altogether. When possible, choose organic products from pasture-raised cows. Listen to your body's cues regarding whether dairy is beneficial or detrimental for your individual health.

CHAPTER 14: THE COMPLEX RELATIONSHIP BETWEEN DIETARY CHOLESTEROL AND HEART DISEASE

For decades, dietary cholesterol was believed to play a major role in raising blood cholesterol levels and heart disease risk. However, recent research has painted a more nuanced picture about the relationship between cholesterol in food and heart health. Here, we review some of the key points.

- Dietary cholesterol comes from animal foods like eggs, meat, and dairy. It differs from the cholesterol naturally produced by the liver.

- While dietary cholesterol can impact blood cholesterol levels, for most people the effect is relatively small compared to saturated fats.

- Newer research indicates dietary cholesterol has a marginal impact on heart disease risk for otherwise healthy individuals.

- Limiting processed meats and high-fat dairy appears more important than dietary cholesterol for heart health.

- For those with cardiometabolic conditions like diabetes or hyperlipidemia, limiting dietary cholesterol may provide some benefit.

- Both genetics and the overall composition of the diet influence how dietary cholesterol affects an individual's blood lipids and heart disease risk.

- Statins and other pharmaceutical drugs are often much more effective at lowering high cholesterol levels than just dietary changes alone.

- While dietary cholesterol in moderation likely poses little risk for most, processed meats and high-fat dairy should still be limited as part of an overall heart-healthy diet.

- Individual responses vary based on genetic factors and medical history. Those concerned should have their blood lipids tested and consult their doctor.

- For heart health, the emphasis should be on limiting saturated/trans fats, processed foods, and added sugars rather than just dietary cholesterol alone.

In summary, the relationship between dietary cholesterol and heart disease risk is complex and dependent on numerous factors. While dietary cholesterol restriction may provide modest benefits for some, improving overall diet quality appears more important for most people. As always, it's best to take a personalised approach based on your individual health profile and risk factors.

CHAPTER 15:
A BALANCED PERSPECTIVE ON SOY

Potential Health Benefits and Controversies

Soy foods like tofu, edamame, and tempeh have generated both hype and controversy over their health effects. Here, we provide an evidence-based look at the potential benefits and controversies surrounding soy consumption.

Potential Health Benefits

- Soy provides high-quality vegetarian protein with all essential amino acids.

- Soy foods contain polyunsaturated fats, fibre, vitamins, and minerals.

- Soy may lower LDL ("bad") cholesterol levels, benefiting heart health.

- Consumption of soy early in life may reduce breast cancer risk for some women.

- Soy isoflavones may help relieve menopausal symptoms like hot flashes.

Nutrition And Health Controversies

- Soy contains phytoestrogens. However, they appear to have weak oestrogen-like effects in humans that don't adversely impact health.

- Despite some concerns, most studies find soy does not increase breast cancer risk or impact oestrogen levels in healthy women.

- Soy infant formula remains controversial. While safe for most babies, breastfeeding is ideal. Consult a paediatrician.

- Soy does not appear to lower testosterone in men or negatively impact testicular function. But data on fertility is conflicting.

- Soy allergies do exist and can cause severe reactions in sensitive individuals. However, soy allergies are uncommon overall.

The Bottom Line

Soy foods can be part of a healthy, balanced diet. But as with any food, moderation is key. Consuming soy in place of more processed foods may provide health benefits for many people. However, individuals with soy allergies or certain hormone-dependent conditions should take precautions. As usual, it's best to vary your protein sources and talk to your healthcare provider about what is appropriate for your unique health history.

CHAPTER 16:
10 NATURAL APPROACHES TO ENHANCE TESTOSTERONE LEVELS AFTER 50

As a man crosses the threshold into his 50s, he often experiences a series of shifts in health and vigour. One common alteration is the gradual decline in testosterone levels. While a moderate decrease in testosterone is a natural part of ageing, substantial drops can impact energy, mood, muscle mass, sexual function, and more.

The reassuring news is that there exist innate methods to invigorate your testosterone levels post-50. By making strategic adjustments to your diet and incorporating targeted supplements, you can actively maintain your testosterone at healthful levels as you navigate the ageing process.

Refining Diet For Elevated Testosterone

Your dietary choices wield a significant influence over hormone regulation. Here are some dietary modifications that can effectively stimulate the body's innate testosterone production:

1. Embrace Nutrient-Rich Fats

Foods such as avocados, olive oil, nuts, seeds, and fatty fish provide the building blocks for your body's testosterone production. Aim for around 25-30% of your daily caloric intake to stem from nourishing monounsaturated and polyunsaturated fats.

2. Amplify Vitamin D and Zinc Consumption

Inadequate levels of vitamin D and zinc have shown correlations with diminished testosterone. Bolster these levels by incorporating foods like shellfish, beef, spinach, mushrooms, and fortified products. In some cases, supplementation might be necessary.

3. Curtail Sugar and Processed Carbohydrates

A diet high in sugar and refined carbs can gradually deplete testosterone levels. Scale back on processed foods, baked goods, sugary cereals, beverages, and desserts. Prioritise whole, unprocessed foods.

4. Elevate Protein Intake

Protein delivers essential amino acids that play a pivotal role in testosterone synthesis. Opt for sources such as meat, fish, eggs, nuts, seeds, legumes, and dairy, aiming for a daily intake of 0.5-0.8 grams of protein per pound of body weight.

5. Integrate Cruciferous Vegetables

Broccoli, cabbage, Brussels sprouts, bok choy, and cauliflower contain compounds that may bolster testosterone production.

Aim for 1-2 servings of these vegetables in your daily diet.

Effective Supplementation

Supplementing your diet with specific elements can also contribute to a testosterone boost. Here are five options to consider:

1. Vitamin D and Zinc

Supplementing with forms such as vitamin D3 and zinc gluconate can help you meet your daily requirements for these essential nutrients.

2. D-Aspartic Acid

This amino acid has demonstrated its capacity to elevate testosterone levels in men with deficiencies. A daily intake of 2-3 grams is recommended.

3. Magnesium

Magnesium supports the function of over 300 enzymes and has been linked to heightened testosterone levels. Aim for a daily intake of 400-500 mg, preferring forms like citrate or glycinate.

4. Ginger

Ginger displays potential in enhancing testosterone levels and promoting sperm health. Consider supplementing with 500-1000 mg of ginger daily.

5. Ashwagandha

This Ayurvedic herb is believed to enhance testosterone levels and fertility. An intake of 500-600 mg of extract one to two times per day is suggested.

Upholding a testosterone-friendly lifestyle encompassing dietary adjustments, regular exercise, stress management, and sufficient sleep is crucial for maintaining optimal testosterone levels in your later years. Should low testosterone significantly impact your daily life, consulting a medical professional to discuss potential treatment options is advised.

By thoughtfully incorporating lifestyle adjustments, you can effectively sustain your testosterone at optimal levels beyond 50. Prioritise a nourishing diet, targeted supplementation, and other health-conscious practices to remain vibrant and energetic as you journey through the later stages of life.

CHAPTER 17: MAINTAINING HEALTHY ARTERIES AND BLOOD PRESSURE THROUGH DIET

Heart disease is one of the leading causes of death worldwide. Luckily, there are steps you can take through your diet to promote heart health. Getting adequate amounts of calcium and magnesium from foods can help maintain healthy arteries and normal blood pressure. In this chapter, I'll discuss some of the top food sources of these important minerals.

Calcium And Magnesium For Cardiovascular Health

Calcium and magnesium work together to support several

aspects of cardiovascular health. Calcium is needed for proper contraction of the heart muscle, normal heart rhythm, and blood clotting. Magnesium helps regulate blood pressure by relaxing blood vessels. It's also involved in nerve signalling and muscle contractions, including the heart's rhythm.

Diets low in calcium and magnesium have been associated with increased risk of high blood pressure and atherosclerosis (hardening of the arteries). Getting enough of these minerals through food can help protect long-term heart health. The current daily recommendations are 1,000-1,200mg of calcium and 320-420 mg of magnesium for adults.

Top Dietary Sources Of Calcium

Dairy products are excellent sources of calcium. For example, one cup of milk or yogurt provides about 300mg. Other non-dairy options are also available:

- Kale, broccoli, and Chinese cabbage all supply around 100 mg calcium per cooked cup.

- Fortified cereals, orange juice, soy/almond milk, and tofu are also good sources, providing 200-350mg per cup or serving.

- Sardines and salmon with bones offer large amounts of highly absorbable calcium, with over 300mg in a 3-ounce can.

- Beans, chickpeas, and some nuts and seeds supply smaller amounts that add up.

Magnesium All-Stars

- Green leafy vegetables are magnesium superstars. For instance, a cup of cooked spinach or Swiss chard provides 150-175mg. Here are more top sources:

- Whole grains like oats, brown rice, and quinoa supply around 50-100mg magnesium per cooked cup.

- Nuts and seeds are very rich in magnesium, with 150-250mg per ounce.

- Fish, beans, avocados, bananas, and dark chocolate offer good amounts.

- Magnesium is also added to some fortified breakfast cereals and other foods.

A heart-healthy diet featuring plenty of calcium and magnesium-rich foods can help keep your arteries and blood pressure within healthy ranges. Be sure to aim for the recommended daily amounts by including a variety of these nutrient-dense options. Your heart will thank you!

CHAPTER 18:
APRICOT SEEDS

Throughout history, nature has been a wellspring of remedies and marvels for human health. Among these treasures lies the unassuming apricot seed, often overlooked despite its array of health benefits and intriguing historical background. One of the most compelling assertions surrounding apricot seeds is their potential as a cancer cure. In this chapter, we aims to delve into the health advantages, historical relevance, and current state of research regarding the utilisation of apricot seeds in cancer treatment.

Unveiling the Health Benefits, Historical Significance, and Potential as a Cancer Treatment

Health Benefits Of Apricot Seeds

Apricot seeds, also known as apricot kernels, are the seeds nestled within the pits of apricots. They are replete with nutrients and harbour essential compounds that contribute to overall health. Here are some of the primary health benefits attributed to apricot seeds:

1. Vitamin B17 (Laetrile): Apricot seeds are renowned for their elevated content of vitamin B17, also recognized as laetrile or amygdalin. Laetrile is a naturally occurring compound found in various plants, including apricot seeds. It is often touted for its potential anticancer properties.

2. Antioxidants: Despite their size, these seeds pack a punch in the form of powerful antioxidants like vitamin E. These substances combat oxidative stress and free radicals within the body, playing a crucial role in shielding cells from damage and promoting overall well-being.

3. Digestive Aid: Apricot seeds are a rich source of dietary fibre, which aids in digestion and fosters a healthy gut. A sufficient intake of fibre is associated with a reduced risk of gastrointestinal issues and improved bowel movements.

4. Healthy Fats: These seeds contain monounsaturated fats, which are heart-healthy fats known to lower bad cholesterol levels and decrease the risk of cardiovascular diseases.

5. Immunity Boost: The vitamins and minerals found in apricot seeds, including vitamin C, iron, and zinc, contribute to fortifying the immune system and augmenting the body's capacity to combat infections.

Historical Significance Of Apricot Seeds

The utilisation of apricot seeds for medicinal purposes boasts a rich history dating back centuries. Native to Central Asia, apricot trees (Prunus armeniaca) have played a prominent role in traditional Chinese medicine, where they were employed in the treatment of various maladies such as coughs, asthma, and constipation. Ayurvedic medicine also esteemed the seeds for their purported anti-inflammatory and analgesic properties.

In the early 20th century, the notion of laetrile as a cancer remedy gained traction, particularly in the United States. Primarily sourced from apricot seeds, laetrile was championed as a "natural" cancer cure. However, due to its potential toxicity and limited empirical evidence, the use of laetrile as a cancer treatment remains a subject of intense debate.

Apricot Seeds And Cancer: The Controversy

The contention surrounding the notion that apricot seeds, particularly their laetrile content, can cure cancer has sparked substantial debate. Advocates posit that laetrile, activated by an enzyme within the tumour, can selectively target cancer cells, leading to their destruction. However, scientific substantiation for these claims is currently insufficient.

Numerous studies have been conducted to assess the efficacy of laetrile as a cancer treatment, but results have yielded inconclusive or even negative findings. Both the American

Cancer Society and the Food and Drug Administration (FDA) have cautioned against using laetrile or apricot seeds as a cancer treatment due to potential risks, such as cyanide poisoning, which can occur when laetrile breaks down in the body.

It is imperative to emphasise that there is no substitute for evidence-based cancer treatments, including surgery, chemotherapy, radiation therapy, and immunotherapy. Patients should consistently consult with qualified medical professionals and adhere to their recommendations for the best possible treatment options.

Conclusion

Apricot seeds undoubtedly bestow a multitude of health benefits, supplying essential nutrients and antioxidants to the body. However, while the historical significance of apricot seeds in traditional medicine is intriguing, their employment as a standalone cancer cure is not substantiated by ample scientific evidence.

As research endeavours continue, we may glean further insights into the potential health advantages of apricot seeds and their constituents. For now, it is crucial to approach assertions of miraculous cures with a measure of skepticism and to always rely on evidence-based medical treatments for serious health conditions like cancer. While nature holds immense potential for wellness, our understanding must remain firmly rooted in scientific rigour and safety.

CHAPTER 19:
PROBIOTICS FOR
AN AGEING BRAIN

Do Healthy Bacteria Boost Cognition?

As we grow older, changes in the gut microbiome and decreased cognitive skills often occur in tandem. This has led scientists to hypothesise that maintaining a healthy community of gut bacteria may help preserve cognitive abilities into old age. Emerging research on probiotics suggests these beneficial microorganisms could be a key piece of the puzzle.

The gut microbiome refers to the vast population of bacteria and other microbes that live in the intestines. This complex internal ecosystem plays important roles in nutrient absorption, digestion, metabolism, and immunity. Intriguingly, the gut microbiome also communicates with the brain via the gut-brain axis.

Studies indicate that unhealthy changes in the gut microbiome are linked to inflammation, diminished brain function, and conditions like Alzheimer's disease. Supplementing with probiotics may help counteract these detrimental shifts.

Probiotics are live microorganisms that provide health benefits when consumed. Common probiotic strains are types of bacteria that normally inhabit the human gut. Probiotic foods and supplements replenish healthy gut bacteria to optimise the microbiome.

Research demonstrates that probiotic supplementation can improve markers of cognitive function including memory, learning, and reaction time. For example, a placebo-controlled trial published in Frontiers in Aging Neuroscience found that consuming a multi-strain probiotic for 12 weeks significantly improved cognitive performance in adults over 60 years old.

Experts propose that enhancing the gut microbiome with probiotics may benefit cognition through several pathways. These include reduced inflammation, optimised brain cell signalling, increased production of mood-regulating neurotransmitters, and improved insulin sensitivity.

As life expectancies lengthen, supporting brain health into old age is a major public health goal. Modulating the gut microbiome through probiotic intake represents a promising supplemental approach to maintaining cognitive abilities as we age. Consuming probiotic-rich foods like yogurt, kefir, and fermented vegetables may lend your brainpower a helping hand.

CHAPTER 20: ARTHRITIS AND DIET

Arthritis, a chronic condition characterised by joint inflammation, often leads to discomfort, stiffness, and reduced mobility. While medical interventions and physical therapy play vital roles in symptom management, the impact of diet on alleviating arthritis-related discomfort should not be overlooked. Specifically, certain protein-rich foods have been associated with heightened inflammation and increased symptoms in individuals with arthritis. In this chapter, we will delve into the protein-rich foods to steer clear of for those grappling with arthritis, aiming to potentially enhance their overall well-being.

Avoiding Protein-Rich Foods For Alleviating Arthritis Pain

Steering Clear of Red Meat

Red meat, encompassing beef, lamb, and pork, constitutes a significant protein source in many diets. However, it boasts elevated levels of arachidonic acid, a fatty acid known to trigger the body's inflammatory response. Regular consumption of red meat for arthritis sufferers may result in heightened inflammation and exacerbated joint pain. Opting for leaner cuts or reducing red meat intake can assist in managing arthritis symptoms effectively.

Cautious Approach to Processed Meats

Processed meats like sausages, bacon, and deli meats not only feature high saturated fat content but also often contain additives such as nitrites and nitrates. These compounds can incite inflammation in the body, exacerbating arthritis symptoms. For individuals with arthritis, opting for leaner protein sources like chicken, turkey, or fish is a more beneficial choice.

Mindful Consumption of High-Fat Dairy Products

Full-fat dairy items like whole milk, cheese, and butter are abundant in saturated fats, which have been linked to inflammation and heightened joint pain. While dairy serves as a crucial calcium source, it is imperative for arthritis sufferers to opt for low-fat or non-fat alternatives to mitigate potential inflammatory effects.

Limiting Fried Foods

Fried foods, encompassing items like fried chicken, French fries, and fried snacks, are replete with unhealthy fats that contribute to inflammation. The high cooking temperatures and oils utilised in frying can generate harmful compounds that trigger an immune response. Individuals with arthritis should consider minimising or abstaining from fried foods in their dietary choices.

Exercising Caution with Shellfish

Certain shellfish varieties like shrimp, crab, and lobster boast elevated purine levels, which the body converts into uric acid.

For those prone to gout, a type of arthritis prompted by high uric acid levels, consuming purine-rich foods can lead to painful gout attacks. Individuals with gout-related arthritis should monitor their shellfish intake and consider lower-purine protein alternatives.

Selective Choices with Beans and Legumes

While beans and legumes are generally considered wholesome protein sources, specific varieties may incite inflammation in arthritis sufferers. Lentils, chickpeas, and soybeans are rich in purines, akin to shellfish, and may necessitate moderation or avoidance for individuals with gout-related arthritis. Conversely, other beans like black beans and kidney beans are typically safe options.

Conclusion

Embracing a balanced, anti-inflammatory diet can serve as a valuable complement to medical interventions for individuals grappling with arthritis. Protein is a crucial nutrient, but the sources we choose to consume warrant thoughtful consideration, especially for those contending with arthritis. Steering clear of or limiting specific protein-rich foods, including red meat, processed meats, high-fat dairy, fried foods, and purine-rich shellfish and legumes, may contribute to managing inflammation and alleviating arthritis symptoms.

It is highly recommended to consult with a healthcare professional or a registered dietitian before making significant dietary changes, particularly for individuals with specific dietary requirements or medical conditions. By making informed choices and embracing a healthier eating plan, arthritis sufferers can take charge of their well-being and enhance their overall quality of life.

CHAPTER 21: THE HUMBLE CLOVE

More Than Meets the Eye

The clove is an unassuming little spice that most of us keep tucked away in our spice racks. But beyond adding warmth and complexity to soups, stews, and baked goods, the clove has a long history of uses as a medicinal herb. In this chapter, we'll explore some of the potential benefits of clove, including one of my personal favourites - clove tea.

What is Clove?

Cloves come from the flower buds of the Syzygium aromaticum tree, which is native to Indonesia. Along with nutmeg, cinnamon, and black pepper, clove is one of the most valuable spices in history. In the past, wars were fought and lands conquered over this tiny dried bud.

Cloves have a sweet yet spicy flavour and are rich in compounds like eugenol, acetyl eugenol, beta-caryophyllene, and vanillin. These components give clove its antioxidant, anti-inflammatory, and anaesthetic properties.

Benefits of Clove Tea

Clove tea is a traditional remedy used to treat a variety of ailments. Here are some of the research-backed benefits of clove tea:

- Anti-inflammatory: Compounds in cloves, including eugenol and acetyl eugenol, are potent anti-inflammatory agents that may help reduce inflammation. This can aid inflammatory conditions like arthritis.
- Antioxidant: Clove is rich in antioxidants, which help protect cells against damage from things like free radicals and oxidative stress. This may promote overall health.
- Antimicrobial: Research shows that clove exhibits antimicrobial effects against certain bacteria, viruses, and fungi. Clove tea may help fight off infections.
- Digestive aid: Clove tea appears to stimulate digestive enzymes and promote gastrointestinal health. It may be useful for treating issues like nausea, bloating, and hiccups.
- Oral health: Eugenol in cloves has natural anaesthetic and antiseptic properties. Gargling with clove tea may temporarily relieve toothache pain and oral ulcers.

How to Make Clove Tea

Making a cup of this warming, soothing tea is easy:

- Add 2-3 whole cloves or 1/4 teaspoon ground clove to a cup of hot water
- Let steep for 5-10 minutes
- Strain out the cloves and add honey to taste if desired. Be sure not to give honey to infants under one year old.

You can also add other herbs and spices like cinnamon, black peppercorns, fresh ginger, lemon, and cardamom to complement the clove flavour. Sip your clove tea slowly and enjoy its therapeutic benefits.

A Simple Remedy With A Complex History

The next time you spy that little bottle of cloves in your pantry, think of its rich past and promising future. This humble dried flower bud punches above its weight when it comes to potential wellness applications. So steep yourself a cup of antioxidant-packed, anti-inflammatory clove tea and drink it in its history.

CHAPTER 22: THE LINK BETWEEN VEGETARIAN DIETS AND HEART HEALTH

Heart disease remains the number one cause of mortality worldwide, accounting for over 17 million deaths annually. However, an abundance of research indicates that adopting a vegetarian diet can significantly reduce the risk of developing heart disease and experiencing adverse cardiac events like heart attacks. In this chapter, we will explore the substantial evidence demonstrating the cardiovascular benefits of plant-based diets.

What The Research Shows

Numerous large observational studies following thousands of participants have uncovered markedly lower rates of heart disease among vegetarian populations compared to non-vegetarians.

For instance, in the EPIC-Oxford study, researchers followed over 44,000 men and women in the United Kingdom for an average of 11 years. The participants included meat eaters, fish eaters, vegetarians, and vegans. At the study's conclusion, after controlling for influencing factors like physical activity, smoking status, and alcohol consumption, the incidence of heart disease was found to be 32% lower among vegetarians compared to participants who ate meat.

Similarly, in the Adventist Health Study-2 involving over 96,000 men and women, pesco-vegetarians and vegans had a 19% and 25% respectively lower risk of developing heart disease compared to meat eating participants. The reduced risks remained even after adjusting for other lifestyle habits.

In 2019, another major meta-analysis compiled data from nine high-quality cohort studies including over 120,000 participants. Vegetarian diets were associated with a 22% reduced risk of coronary heart disease events like heart attacks compared to non-vegetarians after accounting for confounding variables.

Factors Behind The Cardiovascular Benefits

Several key factors contribute to the apparent cardiovascular benefits of plant-based diets:

Blood Pressure - Vegetarians typically have significantly lower blood pressure levels compared to their meat-eating counterparts. Elevated blood pressure is a primary risk factor for heart attacks, strokes, and other cardiovascular events. The fibre, potassium, antioxidants and plant protein in plant-rich diets enhance blood pressure regulation.

Cholesterol Levels - Multiple studies indicate that vegetarians tend to have markedly lower LDL cholesterol levels. LDL cholesterol accumulates in blood vessel walls and initiates atherosclerosis, the narrowing of arteries that underlies heart attacks and angina. Saturated fats commonly found in meat raise LDL, while fibre and plant sterols in veggies help reduce it.

Metabolic Factors - Vegetarians exhibit lower rates of metabolic syndrome - the combination of high blood sugar, excess body fat around the waist, elevated cholesterol, and hypertension that magnifies heart disease risk. Plant foods help regulate blood sugar, reduce inflammation, and lower heart disease risk factors.

Beyond these factors, some research indicates adhering to a lacto-ovo vegetarian or vegan diet reduces the thickness of the carotid arteries supplying the brain. Thinner carotid arterial walls may allow expanded passage of blood flow and oxygen. Vegetarians also have enhanced peripheral arterial function which influences the diameter of blood vessels and impacts cardiovascular health.

The Takeaway

In summary, embracing a vegetarian dietary pattern appears to provide tremendous advantages when it comes to maintaining a healthy heart and avoiding America's number one killer. Choosing to emphasise whole plant foods over meat seems to beneficially influence numerous risk factors like elevated blood pressure, high cholesterol, and heightened inflammation that underpin heart attacks and angina pectoris.

For those concerned about optimising cardiovascular wellness, switching to a vegetarian diet absent of all meat or a mostly plant-based Mediterranean style diet could be one of the most effective nutritional changes you implement. That said, any shift towards incorporating more fruits, vegetables, whole grains, nuts, seeds, and legumes into your eating routine can provide incremental protective effects.

As with any major dietary switch, be sure to seek guidance from a knowledgeable physician or registered dietitian to ensure adequate intake of protein, iron, zinc, vitamin B12 and other essential nutrients. With some planning and adjustments, vegetarian and plant-centric diets can be safe and sustainable for people throughout all phases of life. Your heart will thank you for embracing the wholesome goodness of vegetation!

CHAPTER 23: MANAGING STOMACH ULCERS

Stomach ulcers, also known as gastric ulcers, are painful sores that develop in the lining of the stomach. They can cause discomfort, burning sensations, and even bleeding. While medication plays a crucial role in treating stomach ulcers, lifestyle modifications, including dietary changes, are equally important for managing the condition. In this chapter, we will explore practical ways to manage stomach ulcers and provide a 7-day meal plan to help you make healthier choices.

Managing Stomach Ulcers: Practical Tips And A 7-Day Meal Plan

Understand Your Triggers: Certain foods and beverages can aggravate stomach ulcers and increase discomfort. Common triggers include spicy foods, acidic foods, alcohol, caffeine, and high-fat meals. Keep a food diary to identify which items worsen your symptoms and avoid them.

Opt for a Balanced Diet: A well-balanced diet is essential for managing stomach ulcers. It should include a variety of nutrient-rich foods. Focus on incorporating lean proteins, whole grains, fruits, vegetables, and low-fat dairy products into your meals. These foods are less likely to irritate your stomach and can aid in healing.

Include High-Fibre Foods: Fibre plays a crucial role in maintaining digestive health. It helps regulate bowel movements and prevents constipation, which can worsen ulcer symptoms. Include fibre-rich foods like whole grains, legumes, fruits, and vegetables in your diet. However, if high-fibre foods exacerbate your symptoms, consult with your healthcare provider for personalised advice.

Small, Frequent Meals: Instead of consuming large meals, opt for smaller, more frequent meals throughout the day. Eating smaller portions helps reduce the workload on your digestive system and can alleviate discomfort. Plan your meals and snacks in advance to ensure you have a steady supply of nourishment without overwhelming your stomach.

Avoid Late-Night Eating: Eating too close to bedtime can increase acid production and contribute to acid reflux, making stomach ulcer symptoms worse. Try to finish your last meal or snack at least two to three hours before going to bed. This allows your stomach to empty partially, reducing the risk of acid reflux during the night.

Stay Hydrated: Adequate hydration is essential for overall health and can help manage stomach ulcers. Drink plenty of water throughout the day to keep your body hydrated. Avoid carbonated beverages and acidic juices, as they can aggravate your symptoms. Herbal teas and non-citrus fruit juices are good alternatives.

7-Day Meal Plan:

Day 1:

- Breakfast: Oatmeal topped with sliced bananas and a sprinkle of chia seeds.
- Snack: Greek yogurt with honey and a handful of almonds.
- Lunch: Grilled chicken breast with steamed vegetables and quinoa.
- Snack: Carrot sticks with hummus.
- Dinner: Baked salmon with roasted sweet potatoes and a side salad.
- Dessert: Baked apple slices with a sprinkle of cinnamon.

Day 2:

- Breakfast: Whole grain toast with avocado and poached eggs.
- Snack: Mixed berries with a dollop of Greek yogurt.
- Lunch: Spinach salad with grilled shrimp, cherry tomatoes, and a light vinaigrette.
- Snack: Almond butter on rice cakes.
- Dinner: Turkey meatballs with whole wheat pasta and steamed broccoli.
- Dessert: Fresh melon slices.

Day 3:

- Breakfast: Vegetable omelette with whole grain toast.
- Snack: Celery sticks with almond butter.
- Lunch: Quinoa and black bean salad with a lemon-herb dressing.

- Snack: Trail mix with dried fruits and nuts.
- Dinner: Grilled tofu with stir-fried vegetables and brown rice.
- Dessert: Greek yogurt with a drizzle of honey.

Day 4:

- Breakfast: Overnight chia pudding with mixed berries.
- Snack: Apple slices with a handful of walnuts.
- Lunch: Grilled chicken Caesar salad with whole grain croutons.
- Snack: Cucumber slices with tzatziki dip.
- Dinner: Baked cod with roasted Brussels sprouts and quinoa.
- Dessert: Dark chocolate squares.

Day 5:

- Breakfast: Whole grain cereal with low-fat milk and sliced peaches.
- Snack: Cherry tomatoes with mozzarella cheese.
- Lunch: Lentil soup with a side of whole grain bread.
- Snack: Banana smoothie with almond milk and a dash of cinnamon.
- Dinner: Grilled steak with steamed asparagus and mashed sweet potatoes.
- Dessert: Mixed berry parfait with Greek yogurt.

Day 6:

- Breakfast: Whole grain pancakes topped with fresh berries and a drizzle of maple syrup.
- Snack: Hard-boiled eggs with cherry tomatoes.

- Lunch: Caprese salad with fresh basil, tomatoes, mozzarella, and balsamic glaze.
- Snack: Rice cakes with almond butter and sliced bananas.
- Dinner: Baked chicken breast with roasted vegetables and quinoa.
- Dessert: Grilled pineapple slices with a sprinkle of coconut flakes.

Day 7:

- Breakfast: Vegetable frittata with a side of whole grain toast.
- Snack: Hummus with whole wheat pita bread.
- Lunch: Spinach and strawberry salad with grilled chicken and a light vinaigrette.
- Snack: Mixed nuts and dried fruit.
- Dinner: Grilled shrimp skewers with brown rice and steamed broccoli.
- Dessert: Frozen yogurt with fresh fruit.

Conclusion: Managing stomach ulcers requires a comprehensive approach, including medication and lifestyle modifications. By understanding your triggers, following a balanced diet, and making practical choices, you can alleviate discomfort and support the healing process. Remember to consult with your healthcare provider or a registered dietitian for personalised advice and to ensure the meal plan aligns with your specific needs. By adopting these strategies, you can take control of your stomach ulcers and enjoy a healthier lifestyle.

Here's A 7-Day Meal Plan For Managing Stomach Ulcers With Ingredients Commonly Found In Nigeria:

Day 1:

- Breakfast: Oatmeal cooked with water or low-fat milk, topped with sliced bananas and a sprinkle of ground flaxseeds.
- Snack: Plain yogurt with a drizzle of honey and a handful of peanuts.
- Lunch: Grilled chicken breast with a side of steamed vegetables (such as ugwu or pumpkin leaves) and boiled yam.
- Snack: Watermelon slices.
- Dinner: Baked fish with roasted plantains and a side salad made with cucumber, tomatoes, and lettuce.
- Dessert: Sliced pawpaw (papaya).

Day 2:

- Breakfast: Boiled plantains with scrambled eggs and a side of sliced avocado.
- Snack: Greek yogurt with diced mango.
- Lunch: Efo riro (stewed spinach) with grilled turkey breast and a portion of brown rice.
- Snack: Roasted groundnuts.
- Dinner: Moi moi (steamed bean pudding) made with peeled beans and served with a side of garden egg sauce and boiled sweet potatoes.
- Dessert: Sliced oranges.

Day 3:

- Breakfast: Millet porridge cooked with low-fat milk, cinnamon, and diced apples.
- Snack: Unsweetened Tigernut milk with a small handful of cashew nuts.
- Lunch: Okra soup with grilled fish or chicken and a portion of fufu (made from cassava or yam flour).
- Snack: Sliced cucumbers with a squeeze of lemon juice.
- Dinner: Vegetable stir-fry with grilled beef strips and a side of boiled plantains or brown rice.
- Dessert: Fresh pineapple chunks.

Day 4:

- Breakfast: Whole wheat bread toasted and topped with mashed avocado and sliced tomatoes.
- Snack: African pear (ube) with a handful of almonds.
- Lunch: Chicken pepper soup with boiled yam or unripe plantains.
- Snack: Roasted plantain chips.
- Dinner: Grilled tilapia fish with jollof quinoa (prepared with a tomato-based sauce) and a side salad.
- Dessert: Sliced mangoes.

Day 5:

- Breakfast: Bean porridge (ewa agoyin) made with black-eyed peas, palm oil, and spices, served with a side of boiled plantains.

- Snack: Tigernut cookies (kulikuli).
- Lunch: Banga soup (palm nut soup) with assorted meat and a portion of white rice.
- Snack: Coconut flakes.
- Dinner: Grilled chicken breast with sautéed vegetables (such as green beans, carrots, and bell peppers) and boiled yam.
- Dessert: Sliced watermelon.

Day 6:

- Breakfast: Yam porridge cooked with tomatoes, onions, and bell peppers, served with boiled eggs.
- Snack: Sliced garden egg with peanut butter.
- Lunch: Ogbono soup with fish or chicken and a portion of pounded yam.
- Snack: Roasted corn.
- Dinner: Grilled beef skewers with a side of coleslaw and boiled plantains.
- Dessert: Sliced bananas.

Day 7:

- Breakfast: Nigerian-style scrambled eggs with diced tomatoes, onions, and bell peppers, served with whole wheat bread.
- Snack: Cashew nut milk smoothie with a sprinkle of cinnamon.
- Lunch: Vegetable soup (bitter leaf or ora soup) with goat meat and a portion of semolina or amala.
- Snack: Sliced carrots with hummus.
- Dinner: Grilled mackerel with roasted sweet potatoes and a side salad made with cabbage, tomatoes, and onions.
- Dessert: Sliced guava.

Remember, it's essential to listen to your body and adjust the meal plan according to your specific needs and tolerances. Additionally, consult with a healthcare provider or a registered dietitian for personalised advice and to ensure the meal plan aligns with your individual dietary requirements.

CHAPTER 24: SAFEGUARDING AGAINST COLON CANCER: SCIENCE-BACKED STEPS FOR PREVENTION

Colon cancer need not be an inevitable consequence of aging. Small, daily decisions can wield significant influence in diminishing your risk for this prevalent and potentially serious ailment. Recent studies unveil natural, feasible methods we can employ to help thwart colon cancer, focusing on diet, exercise, and lifestyle - no prescription necessary.

Within this evidence-driven chapter, you'll uncover surprising superfoods for colon cancer prevention, fortified by scientific research. You'll grasp the optimal plant-to-meat ratios for risk reduction, along with intelligent alternatives to processed and red meats. Tailored exercise guidelines designed expressly for colon cancer prevention will demonstrate how staying active can fortify your colon health.

Beyond diet and exercise, we'll delve into lifestyle elements that heighten the risk of colon cancer - and straightforward swaps you can make to sidestep them. Opt for more of this, less of that. Prioritize ample sleep and stress management using proven techniques to help fend off colon cancer. You'll also gain access to the latest screening recommendations to catch issues early, when they are most manageable.

Equip yourself with knowledge and take initiative. Even small, sustainable daily strides can go a long way toward preventing colon cancer. Subtle alterations that bolster your body's innate healing capacities may ultimately be a lifeline. Don't leave your colon health to chance - embark on the journey of colon cancer prevention today!

Colorectal cancer, commonly known as colon cancer, is a prevalent and potentially life-threatening ailment that affects the large intestine. It manifests through the uncontrolled proliferation of abnormal cells in the colon or rectum. While various risk factors contribute to the development of colon cancer, including genetics and age, adopting a healthy lifestyle and implementing practical preventive measures can significantly diminish the risk. In this blog post, we will explore natural methods to reduce the risk of colon cancer and provide actionable strategies for prevention.

Maintaining A Balanced Diet:

A well-rounded diet plays a pivotal role in diminishing the risk of colon cancer. Consider the following dietary recommendations:

a. Amplify Fiber Intake: Integrate high-fiber foods like whole grains, fruits, vegetables, and legumes into your diet. Fiber promotes regular bowel movements and nurtures a thriving digestive system.

b. Restrict Red and Processed Meats: Cut down on red and processed meat consumption as they have been correlated with an elevated risk of colon cancer. Opt instead for lean proteins such as fish and poultry.

c. Embrace Antioxidant-Enriched Foods: Incorporate an array of fruits and vegetables in your diet, as they are replete with antioxidants. These compounds safeguard cells from harm and curtail the risk of cancer.

d. Embrace Wholesome Fats: Elect for wholesome fats like olive oil, avocados, and nuts, which furnish essential nutrients and contribute to overall well-being.

Maintaining A Healthy Weight:

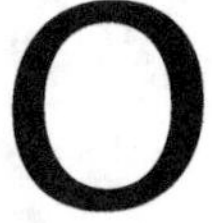

Obesity is linked to an augmented risk of colon cancer. To sustain a healthy weight:

a. Engage in Routine Physical Activity: Strive for at least 150 minutes of moderate-intensity exercise or 75 minutes of vigorous exercise per week. Infuse activities like walking, cycling, or swimming into your routine.

b. Minimize Sedentary Behavior: Steer clear of prolonged periods of sitting and engage in regular movement throughout the day. Take breaks, stretch, and mobilize whenever possible.

c. Regulate Portion Sizes: Exercise prudence with portion sizes to avert excessive calorie intake. Opt for nutrient-dense foods over calorie-dense options.

Lifestyle Adjustments:

Certain lifestyle preferences can contribute to the risk of colon cancer. Adopt the subsequent measures to diminish your risk:

a. Abandon Smoking: Smoking has been associated with an elevated risk of various cancers, including colon cancer. Seek support and resources to quit if you are a smoker.

b. Restrain Alcohol Consumption: Overindulgence in alcohol has been linked to an escalated risk of colon cancer. Moderate your alcohol intake or abstain altogether.

c. Maintain Hydration: Consume a sufficient amount of water throughout the day to preserve proper hydration and foster a healthy digestive system.

Regular Screenings:

Early detection is pivotal in effectively treating colon cancer. Adhere to recommended screening guidelines, typically involving colonoscopies or other screening tests based on your age, family history, and risk factors. Regular screenings aid in identifying precancerous polyps or early-stage colon cancer, heightening the likelihood of successful treatment.

Conclusion:

Diminishing the risk of colon cancer and enacting preventive measures commences with embracing a healthy lifestyle. By making positive choices regarding diet, weight management, physical activity, and steering clear of detrimental habits, you can significantly curtail your risk. Furthermore, regular screenings and medical check-ups allow for early detection and timely intervention, maximizing the prospects of successful treatment. Remember, prevention always trumps cure, and taking proactive steps today can contribute to a future liberated from colon cancer.

CHAPTER 25: CONCLUSION

Conclusion: A Holistic Blueprint For Lifelong Well-Being

As we reach the final chapter of this healthy living guide, I hope you feel equipped, energised and motivated to pursue optimal wellness. More than isolated practices, true health stems from a lifestyle that holistically nurtures body, mind and spirit. It's a journey of progress not perfection. By consistently applying the evidence-based principles we've covered - like eating nourishing whole foods, staying active, reducing stress, getting quality sleep, connecting socially, finding purpose, and seeking professional support when needed - you pave the path for a long, vibrant life.

While every small step matters, the power comes from the cumulative effect of multiple daily choices aligned with your values. Ask yourself - how can I care for this one precious human life I've been given? Your health potential is far greater than you may realise when you commit fully to the process. Get clear on what motivates you, build self-awareness, lean on your support network in the hard moments, and don't forget to celebrate progress. You are worth the investment of time and effort.

Reflect on how far you've already come. Then look ahead - what's one easy change you can make today? Maybe it's taking a short walk, drinking more water, eating an extra vegetable serving or calling a friend. Tiny consistent actions snowball into transformed habits before you know it. The person you'll be a year from now will thank you of today.

To take your health journey to the next level, I encourage ongoing education and discovery. Health insights are constantly evolving. There's always more to learn about nutrition, fitness, stress science, longevity research, alternative therapies and the cutting edge of wellness. Subscribe to reputable sources, take interesting workshops, listen to health podcasts, join local wellness groups and continue reading on emerging topics. Enhance your knowledge so you can optimise your choices. Become your own health advocate.

I also can't stress enough the value of working collaboratively with healthcare professionals throughout your lifespan. Get to know practitioners you trust by being actively involved in your care. Share your health goals transparently so they can provide expert guidance tailored to you. Take advantage of recommended screening tests, wellness visits, bloodwork and monitoring. Early detection of any issues leads to better outcomes. Don't be afraid to ask questions and seek second opinions when needed. You deserve thoughtful, compassionate support.

For optimal health, prioritise loving relationships and a sense of community. We're social creatures wired for connection. Joy is often found in meaningful contribution - volunteering, mentoring others, standing up for causes, expressing your creativity, or sharing hard-earned wisdom. A life well-lived stretches beyond personal gain to enrich the collective whole. When your days have purpose and belonging, inner peace follows.

Remember that true self care also requires self-acceptance - being kind to yourself on the tougher days and loving your body at every size or ability level. We're all perfectly imperfect works in progress. With resilient spirit, you will shine. Don't compare yourself to others or get mired in self-criticism if you have temporary setbacks. Every day is a chance to start fresh.

My hope is that through this book, you've been empowered to take charge of your health in a sustainable, flexible way. Wellness is more than obligatory drudgery - it's learning the keys to being fully alive. Discover activities, foods and lifestyle tweaks that make you come alive too. See this not as a rigid prescription but a jumping off point to keep blossoming into your healthiest, happiest self through the decades ahead. That glowing vitality that resides inside you is ready to be unleashed. Go out and thrive! I'm rooting for your success.

In health and wellness,
Larry Allen

BOOKS BY THIS AUTHOR

Journey To Promethea: A Tale Of Two Minds

Journey to Promethea
Imagine a world divided. A world of vast disparities in rights, wealth, and opportunity. Where factors of birth and status dictate the course of one's entire life. Picture the injustice, the structural barriers that suppress human potential.

The realm of Promethea was such a world - until bold voices dared imagine something better. This is the story of their struggle.

It began small, in the heart of one marginalised boy. Olu, denied the chance to rise beyond his lowly station. But through a spark of education, his mind ignited.

If knowledge was power, then why not enlighten all minds, empower all voices? From this simple question, a movement for justice grew.

Olu and fellow seekers faced suspicion, then defiance, from those clinging to entrenched power. But the people's conscience had awakened. The light of change could not be extinguished.

Generation by generation, progress marched on. With cascading waves of reform, Promethea gradually transformed itself. From classism to inclusion, exploitations to ethics, barriers to bounty shared by all.

Utopia bloomed, an ideal but fragile flower. Early victory cultivated complacency, allowing injustice to creep insidiously back. But voices like Olu's persisted, reminding the people of hard lessons once learned.

Promethea's light had to shine ever brighter, so its glow could uplift other worlds still lost in darkness. This was now their destiny and burden - to herald freedom's possibility, until inequality existed no more.

The Ephemeral Journey Of Mary

Ephemeral Footsteps

What is life but a series of moments - some brilliant as sunshine, others shrouded in shadow, all ephemeral as grains of sand slipping through our fingers? We spend our fleeting time here searching for meaning, connection, purpose. We love, we lose, we learn, and hopefully leave a lasting imprint on the world as we hurry to our horizons.

This book chronicles the journey of a single life, from first tentative steps to final fading footprints. But within one person's story, you may glimpse something universal. We all walk different paths, but embark on the same essential human trek.

The journey begins, as all do, with a child full of innocence and eagerness for the road ahead. She does not yet grasp the brevity of her days or the trials she will come to face. For now, life is wonder, exploration, dreams unlimited by reality.

Like most, this child will encounter crossroads that alter her course. She will discover the ecstasies of love and the agonies of grief. Her spirit will be tested by storms, but emerge more resilient. Joy will be found in the simple moments - a flower unfurling, the laughter of friends, the embrace of family.

As the seasons shift and time flows by, she will reflect on all she has gained and lost. When her final page approaches, she will reckon with life's meaning and all that waits beyond the horizon.

Her story, though unique, reflects our shared human experience. Its joys are our joys, its sorrows our sorrows. Within these pages await glimpses of your own journey. Let her ephemeral footsteps guide you to reflect on the significance of your own.

For in the end, that is the purpose of this book - to illuminate the poignancy of our fragile lives. To inspire us to walk gently yet courageously through all life gives. And to savour each ephemeral moment before our footprints, like waves upon the sand, are inevitably washed away on time's shore.

Whispers Of Timeless Wisdom

Welcome to "Whispers of Wisdom," a collection of inspirational and thought-provoking quotes that have resonated across cultures and eras. Within these pages, you will find words that uplift the spirit, ignite curiosity, and compel us to reflect deeply on the human experience.

This treasury of quotes traverses centuries, from ancient philosophers to modern visionaries, capturing glimpses of insight on topics ranging from courage, leadership, and self-discovery to love, purpose, and our place in the universe. While the context around these words has shifted over time, their essence continues to ring true.

As you immerse yourself in these whispers of wisdom, may you be filled with inspiration to live your life more fully. May the thoughts shared light your way when the path seems unclear and renew your spirit when challenges arise. For it is often in our darkest moments that words of hope, empathy and encouragement can make the greatest difference.

While some quotes provide clear steps forward, others simply give language to emotions we know to be true but struggle to express. Whatever form they take, these diverse perspectives are bound by a faith in human potential. Though the future remains a mystery, we walk into it emboldened by those who have peered into the unknown before us.

I invite you to quiet your mind as you turn each page. Absorb the insights that speak to you most, then carry them with you through the tapestry of your days. Return to these words when you feel adrift and when your faith needs rekindling. Share them to spark inspiration in others when the opportunity arises. For that is how whispers become wisdom, illuminating our way forward as one human family.

Unearthing The Mother Wound

What is Mother's wound

The term "Mother's wound" is often used in the field of psychology to describe the emotional pain and trauma that can arise from a difficult or disrupted relationship with one's mother. This can occur in many different forms, including neglect, abandonment, abuse, or simply a lack of emotional connection or atonement.

The concept of the Mother's wound was first popularised by the psychologist Dr. Janice Webb in her book "Running on Empty: Overcome Your Childhood Emotional Neglect," in which she describes how a lack of emotional validation and support from one's mother can lead to a sense of emptiness, disconnection, and low self-worth in adulthood.

It's important to note that the Mother's wound is not meant to be a blanket statement about all mothers or to place blame on any one individual. Rather, it is a recognition of the fact that our early relationships with our caregivers can have a profound impact on our emotional development and well-being.

Working through the Mother's wound often involves exploring and processing the complex emotions and experiences associated with this early relationship, and learning to cultivate self-compassion and self-validation.

Understanding the Mother's wound involves exploring and processing the emotions and experiences associated with a difficult or disrupted relationship with one's mother. Here are some steps you can take to gain a deeper understanding of the Mother's wound:

Nature's Pharmacy Meal Plan

Natures Pharmacy Meal Plan: Seven-day meal planner for a healthy diet typically includes a variety of nutrient-dense foods such as whole grains, fruits, vegetables, lean proteins, and healthy fats. The aim is to create a balanced diet that meets the nutritional needs of the individual while supporting overall health and wellbeing. Additionally, the meal plan may include suggestions for meal preparation and cooking techniques to ensure the meals are both healthy and delicious. This book is a comprehensive guide to healthy eating habits.
Contents Includes:
Plant-based seven days meal planner,
Protein Rich seven days meal planner.
Seven-days meal plan that focuses on protein-rich fruits and vegetables.
Seven-day meal planner for a low-salt diet that's also suitable for people with high blood pressure.
Seven-day meal planner for people with diabetes: Seven-day

meal planner for people who have survived a stroke.
Seven-day meal planner for prostate health.
Seven-day meal planner for people with gout:
Seven-day meal planner for people with eczema